Strength and Vitality: Ageless Fitness for Seniors

Unlock Your Potential With Simple, Effective Workouts

Kathryn Rafalowski MSN, RN

© **Copyright 2024 - All rights reserved.**

The content contained within this book may not be reproduced, duplicated or transmitted without direct written permission from the author or the publisher.

Under no circumstances will any blame or legal responsibility be held against the publisher, or author, for any damages, reparation, or monetary loss due to the information contained within this book, either directly or indirectly.

Legal Notice:

This book is copyright protected. It is only for personal use. You cannot amend, distribute, sell, use, quote or paraphrase any part, or the content within this book, without the consent of the author or publisher.

Disclaimer Notice:

Please note the information contained within this document is for educational and entertainment purposes only. All effort has been executed to present accurate, up to date, reliable, complete information. No warranties of any kind are declared or implied. Readers acknowledge that the author is not engaged in the rendering of legal, financial, medical or professional advice. The content within this book has been derived from various sources. Please consult a licensed professional before attempting any techniques outlined in this book.

By reading this document, the reader agrees that under no circumstances is the author responsible for any losses, direct or indirect, that are incurred as a result of the use of the information contained within this document, including, but not limited to, errors, omissions, or inaccuracies.

Table of Contents

INTRODUCTION 1

CHAPTER 1: KNOW THY BODY 5
   THE AGE-DEFYING ANATOMY LESSON 5
      Meet the Heart 6
      Your Lungs 6
      Your Endocrine System 7
      The Nervous System 7
      Musculoskeletal System 7
   CHANGES IN MUSCLE AND BONE DENSITY 8
   THE IMPORTANCE OF BALANCE AND STABILITY 9
   HEALTH HICCUPS AND EXERCISE FIXES 10
      Osteoporosis and Osteoarthritis 10
      Sarcopenia 11
      Alzheimer's Disease and Dementia 11
      Depression 11
      Diabetes 12
      Coronary Heart Disease 12
      Obesity 12
      High Cholesterol 13
      Hypertension or High Blood Pressure 13
   KEY EXERCISE PROGRAMMING TIPS FOR OLDER ADULTS 13
      Low-Intensity Cardio 14
      Focus on Flexibility 14
      High-Intensity Interval Training 14
      Eccentric Exercises 15
      Rate Of Perceived Exertion 15
      Talk Test 15
      Medication 16
   BALANCE AND STABILITY EXERCISES 16
      Feet Apart Balance Exercise 16
      Feet Together Balance Exercise 16
      Semi-Tandem Stance Balance Exercise 17
      Tandem Stance Balance Exercise 17
      Single Leg Stance Exercise 18
      Toe Stands 18
      Rock the Boat 19

Weight Shifts	19
Tight Rope Walk	20
Flamingo Stand	20
Tree Pose	21
Heel to Toe Walk	21
Key Takeaways	22

CHAPTER 2: READY, SET, GO! 23

PAR-Q	23
How Fit and Strong Are You Now?	25
Exercise Safety	28
Listen to Your Body	28
When to Stop Exercising	29
Goal-Setting: Your Personal Everest	30
Getting Motivated	30
Starting Your Journey	30
Adopting Your Program	30
Staying on Track	31
Setting Realistic and Achievable Goals	31
Eliminating Obstacles	33
Home Gym Hacks: Essentials Without the Fuss	34
Create a Budget	34
Invest in Multitasking Equipment First	34
Buy Second-Hand Equipment	35
Create a Dedicated Workout Space	35
Be Aware of Your Surroundings	35
Tidy Up Afterwards	35
Invest in Adequate Storage	36
Limit Distractions	36
Do Not Workout Alone	36
Key Takeaways	36

CHAPTER 3: WARM-UP WONDERS 39

The Warm-up Wizardry	39
The Science Behind Warming Up	39
Easy Peasy Warm-up Moves	40
Gentle Aerobic Warm-Ups	40
Gentle Warm-up Exercises	40
Quick and Easy Warm-up Routine	50
Upper Body Warm-up	50
Lower Body Warm-up	52
Full Body Warm-up	54

CHAPTER 4: PUMP IT UP—STRENGTH TRAINING 59

THE IMPACT OF STRENGTH TRAINING ON COGNITIVE FUNCTION 60
- *The Connection Between Exercise and Mental Health* 61
- *Research Supporting Exercise as a Mental Health Intervention* 61
- *Upper Body Boosters* 62
- *Lower Body Lifters* 68
- *Core Crusaders* 78
- *Full Body Fitness* 84

KEY TAKEAWAYS 89

CHAPTER 5: COOL DOWN LIKE A PRO 91

REDUCING DELAYED ONSET MUSCLE SORENESS (DOMS) 91
PROVIDING STRESS RELIEF 92
GRADUALLY LOWERING YOUR HEART RATE 92
DECREASING THE RISK OF INJURY 93
IMPROVING FLEXIBILITY 93
PREVENTING BLOOD POOLING 94
STRETCH IT OUT: FLEXIBILITY, FUN 94
- *Neck Extension Stretch* 94
- *Neck Flexion Stretch* 94
- *Neck Rotation Stretch* 95
- *Levator Scapula Stretch* 95
- *Neck Side Stretch* 96
- *Thoracic Rotation Stretch* 97
- *Shoulder and Arm Overhead Stretch* 97
- *Upper Arm and Shoulder Stretch* 97
- *Chest Stretch* 98
- *Hamstring Stretch* 98
- *Calf Stretch* 99
- *Hip Flexion Stretch* 100
- *Hip Lateral Rotation Stretch* 100
- *Lumbar Flexion Stretch* 101
- *Lumbar Side Stretch* 101

YOGA COOL-DOWN 102
- *Cobblers Pose* 102
- *Sphinx Pose* 102
- *High Alter Side Lean* 103
- *Torso Circles* 104
- *Cat/Cow* 104
- *Warrior Pose I* 105
- *Warrior II* 106
- *Childs Pose* 107

BREATHE EASY: RELAXATION TECHNIQUES 107

    Pursed Lip Breathing *107*
    Diaphragmatic Breathing *108*
    Lion's Breathe *109*
    Alternate Nostril Breathing *110*
    Equal Breathing *110*
    Sitali Breathing *111*
    Humming Bee Breath *112*
  Key Takeaways 112

CHAPTER 6: BEGINNER'S LUCK 115

  15-Minute Lower Body Workout 115
    Warm-up *115*
    The Workout *117*
    Cool-Down *118*
  15-Minute Upper Body Workout 120
    Warm-up *120*
    The Workout *121*
    Cool-Down *123*
  15-Minute Full-Body Workout 124
    Warm-up *124*
    The Workout *126*
    Cool-Down *128*

CHAPTER 7: MIDWAY MARVELS 131

  30-Minute Lower Body Workout 131
    Warm-up *131*
    The Workout *132*
    Cool-Down *136*
  30-Minute Upper Body Workout 138
    Warm-up *138*
    The Workout *140*
    Cool-Down *143*
  30-Minute Full-Body Workout 145
    Warm-Up *145*
    The Workout *147*
    Cool-Down *151*

CHAPTER 8: ADVANCED ACES 153

  45-Minute Upper Body Workout 153
    Warm-up *153*
    The Workout *156*
    HIIT Workout *158*
    Cool-Down *158*
  45-Minute Lower Body Workout 161

Warm-up *161*
The Workout *162*
HIIT Workout *165*
Cool Down *166*
45-Minute Full-Body Workout 167
Warm-up *167*
The Workout *169*
Cool-Down *173*

CHAPTER 9: NIFTY NUTRITION 175

Calories and Macronutrients 175
Protein *176*
Carbohydrates *178*
Fats *179*
Simple, Tasty Treats 181
Breakfast *181*
Lunch *185*
Dinner *189*
Key Takeaways 194

CONCLUSION..197

REFERENCES..199

Introduction

We are so fortunate to be aging. I know this is not the most common way to look at getting older, but I do truly believe this. As we age, our lives improve in a variety of ways and reasons. We have a greater sense of self and are more comfortable with who we are. We have a deeper desire to connect and have the means to grow these connections, and we have many years of past experiences to draw on that help us make decisions.

Sure, we are also physically getting older, which means more aches and pains, a greater risk of illness and cognitive dysfunction. Still, it is time that we squash these stereotypical narratives about aging and instead look at things more positively. After all, this kind of mindset provides us the motivation to keep on living vibrant lives, allowing nothing to hold us back.

But you know this because you have this book in your hands. You know that you are entering an exciting chapter of your life, and you are not ready to slow down, no matter what society may say about getting older. So you are getting ready.

Strength training is your golden ticket to a happier and full life as you get older. Whether you are inactive or only mildly active at the moment, this book is for you and will help you grow stronger, healthier, more active, and more independent.

I know that it can be overwhelming when looking to start an exercise program, no matter how important we know that it is for our health and wellbeing. There is a lot of information out there, and it can be hard to sift through it all. You may also be wary of safety and whether or not a specific program is suitable for you, or you may even just have problems sticking to one.

This book will cut through all the noise and help you create a safe, simple, and highly effective exercise program based on the principles of strength training, which will help you:

- build strength

- improve and maintain bone density

- improve and maintain muscle mass

- improve balance, coordination, and mobility

- reduce your risk of falling

- maintain your independence

According to research from Seguin and Nelson (2003), additional benefits of strength training include a reduction in signs and symptoms of chronic diseases such as heart disease, arthritis, and type 2 diabetes. It can also improve sleep and reduce depression. The effects that it has in reducing the signs and symptoms of various diseases have been well studied. For those of you suffering from arthritis, it can reduce pain and swelling, plus it increases mobility and strength. It helps improve glycemic control in diabetics. It can help those with osteoporosis by maintaining bone density and reducing the risk of falls—strength training has a positive effect on lipid profiles, which improves our cardiovascular function. If you suffer from back pain, you may find that it alleviates pain as it makes your muscles stronger.

These are just the physical benefits, and when it comes to mental benefits, there are many to be had as well. Strength training can increase your self-confidence, boost self-esteem, and improve your overall mental well-being.

We are so fortunate to live in an age where we have such easy access to so much information. But this can be a blessing and curse as we find that there is a lot of noise out there, a lot of noise out there about strength training and exercise in general that can be misleading or fear-mongering, especially when it focuses on exercise for seniors.

The first misconception about aging, in general, is that it signals a decline in physical and mental capabilities. Like I said earlier, this does not have to be the story that you are telling yourself and others.

Of course, certain diseases are more common as we get older, but this does not automatically mean that we are destined for poor health. In fact, with the right preventative measures in place, such as healthy eating, exercising, and managing stress, we can live full and vibrant lives with a reduced risk of chronic disease or injuries later in life.

Many people also believe that it may be too late to start exercising. It is never too late to start exercising and anything new you add to your routine is going to improve your health and fitness, even if it is a 10-minute daily walk. Every tiny bit of exercise will add to your longevity and provide incredible benefits both physically and mentally.

This book is going to provide you with all the tools you need to begin or restart your health and fitness journey. From learning about your body and how to set goals to constructing warm-up routines and managing your nutrition, you will have a thorough roadmap to follow.

Let's go!

Chapter 1:

Know Thy Body

One thing that is guaranteed in this life is that nothing remains the same. Our bodies are no different; we are constantly changing from the moment we are born and I find this fascinating.

This chapter is going to give you a brief and very simple anatomy lesson where we will look at the various muscles in our bodies and what they are responsible for when it comes to movement. We will look at why it is important for us to continuously work on our balance and stability.

We will explore the common health issues that we need to keep an eye out for as we get older and how we could work around any issues that may prevent us from performing certain exercises because of these.

We will then wrap up this chapter with various balance and stability exercises that you can begin to use as you start your health and fitness journey.

The Age-Defying Anatomy Lesson

I believe that once we are aware of the different systems in our bodies and how they work, we will develop a deeper appreciation for the exercises that help them do their jobs. This knowledge can give us meaning and motivation to exercise as we become familiar with the reasons why consistent movement is so important for us to keep healthy and feel good as we get older.

Our bodies consist of three types of muscles: skeletal, cardiac, and smooth. Skeletal muscles are attached to our bones and tendons. These muscles help us move voluntarily and quickly. Our cardiac muscles are found only in the heart and they work involuntarily and at a moderate speed to keep our heart beating. Finally, smooth muscles, found in hollow organs and blood vessels, work slowly and involuntarily to control functions like digestion and blood flow.

We also have various systems, such as the circulatory system, hematologic system, endocrine system, nervous system, gastrointestinal system, skeletal system, and reproductive system.

We are going to begin by looking at the important muscle in our body, our heart.

Meet the Heart

Our heart is situated between our lungs and within our ribcage. Our ribcage offers it protection. Our heart can be considered a powerful pump, and it pumps blood throughout our bodies. As it moves the blood around our bodies, it also delivers oxygen and nutrients to cells and removes waste (Khan Academy, 2008).

Your heart is about the size of your fist, and it is continuously pumping blood around your body.

Your Lungs

When we breathe in and out, the air travels in through our nose or mouth, down through our throat, through our Adam's apple or voice box, and into the lungs. It is then exhaled back out again.

Your lungs look like an upside-down tree and consist of tiny sacs called alveoli, this is which the air is directed.

Oxygen from the air enters the bloodstream, while waste carbon dioxide exits into the alveoli and is exhaled. As you are aware, breathing is vital for our survival.

Your Endocrine System

The endocrine system is made up of glands that make hormones which carry messages from one cell to another. This means that it influences every cell, organ, and function of our bodies.

It releases and regulates the hormones in our bloodstream. These hormones are responsible for mood, growth and development, the way our organs work, metabolism, and reproduction.

The Nervous System

Your nervous system performs two types of essential functions. The basic functions include automatic responses, such as reflexes, motor control, and sensory detection. The higher functions involve consciousness, emotions, and cognition.

Musculoskeletal System

Our bodies are made up of three different types of muscles: skeletal, cardiac, and smooth. We are going to focus on our skeletal muscles, which are attached to our bones and our tendons, as these are the muscles that help us move and are the most effective by exercise.

To keep these systems functioning optimally, you need to focus on healthy habits such as stress reduction, healthy eating, and, of course, exercise. A consistent exercise routine can help keep all these systems working as they should and help reduce your risks of developing any diseases that might compromise them.

Changes in Muscle and Bone Density

With aging, there come about changes in our muscles and bones. We tend to find it harder to hold on to our muscle mass and bone density, and we tend to lose these over time.

Let's first look at what happens to our bones as we get older. As the years progress, we start to lose bone mass and bone density. This is especially true for women as they reach menopause and their hormones start to change.

As we lose calcium and other minerals, our bones become brittle and weak, which means that they become easier to break and harder to heal. We are also more prone to compression fractures, which can be painful.

There is a decrease the fluids within our joints, which makes them stiffer and less flexible. This may result in cartilage problems as the cartilage begins to rub against the bone and wear away. We may find that minerals also start to deposit in our joints, which makes movement more uncomfortable. This is known as calcification (Mount Sinai, 2017).

As we get older, other degenerative changes occur, particularly in our hips and knees, and we tend to begin losing cartilage in these areas. This also occurs in our fingers, and we find that our bones thicken slightly; this swelling in our bones, known as osteophytes, is more common among women (Mount Sinai, 2017).

Along with changes in our bone density and mass, we also see changes in our muscles. As we get older, our lean body mass decreases as we lose tissue. This can begin to occur as early as our 30s.

As our muscles lose tone, they contract less, and many become more rigid. When we lose our muscle, it becomes more difficult to replace, or it is replaced by fibrous tissue instead.

The effect of these changes in our bones and muscles can lead to other issues.

Our bones become more brittle, and it is easier for them to break. We become shorter than our spine and trunk shrink; this also results in posture changes, and we may find ourselves hunching or stooping. Our necks may tilt, our shoulders narrow, and our pelvises become wider. Additionally, our gait may change, and walking along with other movements becomes harder.

With the loss of muscle, we also lose strength and become weaker.

The good news? We can reduce the risks by moving. Exercise is the answer.

The Importance of Balance and Stability

As we get older, changes in our physiology can result in us becoming more unstable and unbalanced. There are numerous reasons why this happens, ranging from changes in our bones and muscles, as explained above, to changes in our eyesight and hearing.

Balance is the ability to control our body position, whether we are standing or sitting still or moving.

We need to maintain our balance and stability because they allow us to live full lives and maintain our independence as we age. We need good balance to do just about anything, including simple tasks that we take for granted, such as walking, stepping over obstacles, getting out of a chair, and leaning over to tie our shoes. We also need to have good balance to ensure we can successfully navigate rough or uneven surfaces or if we need to shift direction while walking.

Our balance is dependent on three main systems:

- visual
- vestibular
- somatosensory

Our visual system comprises our eyes, which perceive direction and motion; our vestibular system is our inner ear, which helps monitor motions and give us orientation cues and finally, the somatosensory system refers to the feedback we get from our joints in our ankles, knees, spine, and neck which tell us where our body is in space.

Health Hiccups and Exercise Fixes

We become more susceptible to certain ailments as we get older. We have discussed the changes in our bone density and muscles, and these are two areas where we see the prevalence of two specific health conditions. They are osteoporosis and sarcopenia. We also see increased risk in chronic conditions such as heart disease, dementia, type 2 diabetes, arthritis, and cancer.

The good news? Exercise can help reduce your risks and symptoms of these diseases.

Osteoporosis and Osteoarthritis

Osteoporosis is characterized by the weakening of our bones. As we get older, our bones slowly begin to lose calcium and other minerals that keep them strong.

These minerals keep our bones strong, but as we lose them over time, our bones become weak, brittle, and more prone to fracturing and breaking. The problem here is that there are no symptoms, and without a bone density scan, you would not know if you had osteoporosis.

Osteoarthritis affects the cartilage in our joints. Cartlidge cushions your joints and, as you get older, the cushion wears down, which can expose the bones. Pain arises when the bones rub against each other because of the lack of cushioning. You are more likely to suffer from osteoarthritis if you have a previous joint injury or if you are overweight.

Sarcopenia

The medical term for muscle loss that occurs when we get older is sarcopenia. On average, we lose 3% of our muscle mass a year once we pass middle age (Thorpe, 2017). You may feel weaker, have difficulty lifting objects, be more fatigued, and find activities such as walking become more challenging. You may also be losing weight unintentionally.

There are ways to prevent this, which include exercising regularly, specifically resistance training. A well-balanced diet that focuses on an adequate protein intake also ensures that you maintain muscle mass and keep your strength.

Alzheimer's Disease and Dementia

This disease causes memory loss and other cognitive problems, such as difficulty thinking or problem-solving. This can affect daily life.

Although you are more at risk of Alzheimer's and Dementia based on your age, family history, and genetics, there are certain things that you can do to help reduce the onset of these diseases. One of them is exercise, and the other two are sleep and good nutrition National Council on Aging (2024).

Depression

As we go through the normal process of aging, we find that our lives change, and we might have a more difficult time dealing with these changes. Depression can occur when we do not have the coping mechanisms to deal with and manage these mental shifts.

Depression is characterized by sadness, pessimism, hopelessness, fatigue, difficulty making decisions, changes in appetite, a loss of interest in activities, and more.

Exercise helps by improving your mood. When you exercise, you release endorphins and brain chemicals that help you feel good. This can result in an increase in self-confidence and self-worth as you meet your goals and improve your physical appearance. Exercise can also help you make social connections by interacting with others at the gym or in group classes (National Council on Aging, 2024).

If you feel you need professional help, please reach out to a healthcare provider.

Diabetes

Diabetes occurs when your body does not process insulin effectively or does not produce enough insulin (National Council on Aging, 2024).

Insulin helps us get our energy from food and distribute it throughout our body. If this does not happen properly, our blood sugar will rise. Exercise, even for as little as 30 minutes a day, can help keep these levels in check.

Coronary Heart Disease

Also known as Ischemic heart disease, this is a condition that is caused by a build-up of plaque. As the plaque builds up, the arteries in our hearts narrow, which makes blood flow to our hearts difficult. Blood flow decreases, and other complications can arise, such as blood clots, angina, or a heart attack (National Council on Aging, 2024).

Regular cardio exercises can help reduce your risk of coronary heart disease.

Obesity

Changes in our lifestyle, including a reduction in activity and poor eating habits, can result in obesity.

High Cholesterol

High cholesterol occurs when your body has too many bad fats, known as lipids. These fats can clog our arteries and lead to poor heart health.

Hypertension or High Blood Pressure

Hypertension is a condition that is related to blood flow from your heart and how your arteries move that blood around your body.

If your heart pumps out a lot of blood and your arteries are narrowed and resist this flow, you will have high blood pressure. High blood pressure usually has no symptoms and can be undetected for years.

All of these common diseases and ailments can be managed with exercise. The Centers for Disease Control and Prevention advises that people older than 65 years should be performing aerobic, muscle-strengthening, and balance activities each week.

Aerobic physical activity would be at least 150 minutes of moderate-intensity cardio. You could split this up into five 30-minute sessions a week. This could be 30 minutes a day, five days a week.

Alternatively, you could aim for 75 minutes of vigorous-intensity activity or even a combination of both.

It is also recommended that you perform at least 2 days of strength-building activity along with balance exercises.

Key Exercise Programming Tips for Older Adults

Exercise can be adapted and modified based on your specific needs. If you have certain ailments or injuries, you can adapt almost any program to accommodate you. There are also so many different ways to get healthy that you are bound to find something that you enjoy and that works for your lifestyle. From walking or weightlifting to swimming or chair yoga, there is a fitness routine for anyone.

There are some basic recommendations for older adults who are looking to start exercising. Let's take a look at them.

Low-Intensity Cardio

If you suffer from osteoporosis or arthritis, you may find that high-impact activity such as running may be uncomfortable. If this is the case, swap out this cardio for rowing, swimming, cycling, spinning, or water aerobics.

Focus on Flexibility

Flexibility decreases with age and activity, and as we get older, we need to make sure that we are encouraging elasticity and mobility. Reduction is our flexibility can hinder our ability to perform daily tasks and take away from our independence.

You should finish off your exercise sessions with a cool down that incorporates stretching, which will help improve your flexibility.

High-Intensity Interval Training

High-Intensity Interval Training (HIIT) is an exercise routine that alternates between short bursts of intense activity and less intense recovery periods.

This training method is designed to improve cardiovascular fitness, burn fat, and build endurance in a relatively short amount of time. HIIT can be applied to various forms of exercise, including running, cycling, and bodyweight workouts.

The key is to push yourself to your maximum effort during the high-intensity intervals, followed by a period of rest or lower intensity.

If you do incorporate HIIT into your workout program, it is advisable to ensure you have enough rest days between the sessions. The recommendation to optimize recovery is to have 5 days between each session (ACE Fitness, n.d.).

Eccentric Exercises

Eccentric exercises are movements that focus on the lengthening phase of a muscle contraction. During these exercises, the muscle is actively lengthening while it is under tension. For example, when you're slowly lowering a weight during a biceps curl, the biceps undergoes an eccentric contraction as it lengthens while you control the descent of the weight. Eccentric exercises are often used to improve strength, increase muscle mass, and enhance flexibility, and they can be effective for rehabilitation purposes as well. This type of training is beneficial for improving muscle and reducing the risk of injury.

Rate Of Perceived Exertion

Most conventional strength programs base their working weights on 1 Rep Max's, and while this is a great way to get stronger and build muscles as we get older, it is advisable to rather use RPE. Performing at maximal capacity as required when using a 1-RM may not be advised for older adults due to possible moderate to high-risk issues.

Talk Test

When determining the intensity of an exercise, you should use the talk test as a guide. This is a very simple way to gauge how hard you are exerting yourself by paying attention to your ability to talk while exercising.

The harder you are exercising, the harder it will be to talk.

Medication

Many of us may be using medication in our day-to-day lives, and we need to consider this when exercising. The most common medications that are prescribed are those for high cholesterol, hypertension, type 2 diabetes, and cardiovascular disease, and we need to be aware of how they interact with exercise.

Balance and Stability Exercises

Feet Apart Balance Exercise

1. Start by standing up tall next to a chair. The chair will help you keep stable and balanced.

2. Your feet should be positioned just underneath your hips.

3. Stay in this position for as long as you feel comfortable, and if you are unable to keep track of how long, you can do so.

If you find this easy, you can make it more challenging by closing your eyes. To progress even further, you can close your eyes and set yourself an amount of time to hold this position. Additionally, you can perform this exercise on an unstable surface, such as a cushion, or you can add a task, such as bouncing a ball.

Feet Together Balance Exercise

1. Start by standing up tall next to a chair. The chair will help you keep stable and balanced.

2. Position your feet as close together as they can go and take your hand off the chair.

3. Stay in this position for as long as you feel comfortable, and if you are unable to keep track of how long, you can do so.

If you find this easy, you can make it more challenging by closing your eyes. To progress even further, you can close your eyes and set yourself an amount of time to hold this position. Additionally, you can perform this exercise on an unstable surface, such as a cushion, or you can add a task such as bouncing a ball.

You can make this task further challenging by standing on the unstable surface with your eyes closed.

Semi-Tandem Stance Balance Exercise

1. Start by standing up tall next to a chair. The chair will help you keep stable and balanced.

2. Position your feet so that one foot is in front of the other foot. Place your big toe alongside the inside arch of the front foot.

3. Stay in this position for as long as directed, and if you are unable to keep track of how long, you can do so.

4. When you have completed the set time, switch feet and repeat on the other side.

If this is too difficult and you feel too unsteady, you can perform this exercise with two chairs, placing one on either side of you. If you find this easy, you can make it more challenging by closing your eyes. Additionally, you can perform this exercise on an unstable surface, such as a cushion, or you can add a task, such as bouncing a ball.

Tandem Stance Balance Exercise

1. Start by standing up tall next to a chair. The chair will help you keep stable and balanced.

2. Position your feet so that one foot is in front of the other foot. Place your big toe of the back foot into the heel of the front foot.

3. Stay in this position for as long as directed, and if you are unable to keep track of how long, you can do so.

4. When you have completed the set time, switch feet and repeat on the other side.

If this is too difficult and you feel too unsteady, you can perform this exercise with two chairs, placing one on either side of you. If you find this easy, you can make it more challenging by closing your eyes. Additionally, you can perform this exercise on an unstable surface, such as a cushion, or you can add a task, such as bouncing a ball.

Single Leg Stance Exercise

1. Start by standing up tall next to a chair. The chair will help you keep stable and balanced.

2. Stand on one leg.

3. Stay in this position for as long as directed, and if you are unable to keep track of how long, you can do so.

If this is too difficult and you feel too unsteady, you can perform this exercise with two chairs, placing one on either side of you. If you find this easy, you can make it more challenging by closing your eyes. Additionally, you can perform this exercise on an unstable surface, such as a cushion, or you can add a task, such as bouncing a ball.

Toe Stands

1. Start by standing up tall next to a chair. The chair will help you keep stable and balanced.

2. Your feet should be positioned just shoulder-width apart.

3. Carefully raise yourself onto the balls of your feet and count to four.

4. Hold this position for two to four seconds. When you have held this for the set amount of time, slowly lower your heels back to the floor while counting to four.

5. Repeat 10 toe stands for 1 set.

6. Rest for about 1 minute. Then, complete a second set of 10 toe stands.

Rock the Boat

1. Start by standing up tall next to a chair. The chair will help you keep stable and balanced.

2. Your feet should be positioned just underneath your hips.

3. Carefully lift your left for off the floor and bend your knee so that your heel comes up toward your bottom.

4. Hold this position for up to 30 seconds.

5. Swap sides and lift your right foot off the floor.

6. Repeat on each side three more times.

Weight Shifts

1. Start by standing up tall next to a chair. The chair will help you keep stable and balanced.

2. Your feet should be positioned just underneath your hips.

3. Carefully shift your weight onto your right foot while raising your left foot off the ground.

4. Hold this position for up to 30 seconds.

5. Swap sides and lift your right foot off the floor.

6. Repeat on each side three more times.

Tight Rope Walk

1. Raise your arms and extend them out to the sides.

2. Focus your gaze on a fixed point in the distance in front of you and begin to walk in a straight line.

3. Each time you raise your foot, pause with your foot in this raised position for 2 to 3 seconds.

4. Take 20 to 30 steps.

Flamingo Stand

1. Start by standing up tall next to a chair. The chair will help you keep stable and balanced.

2. Your feet should be positioned just underneath your hips.

3. Carefully shift your weight onto your right foot while raising your left foot off the ground and extending it forward.

4. Hold this position for 10 to 15 seconds.

5. Return to the starting position and shake out your legs.

6. Repeat on the same leg three more times.

7. Swap sides and repeat on the other leg.

You can increase the difficulty by reaching your hands toward your extended foot.

Tree Pose

1. Start by standing up tall next to a chair. The chair will help you keep stable and balanced.

2. Place your feet together and arms at your sides.

3. Carefully shift your weight onto your left foot, bend your right knee, and lift your right foot off the ground.

4. Place the sole of your right foot against your left inner thigh, calf, or ankle (but avoid placing it directly on the knee).

5. Place your hands in any comfortable position.

6. Hold for as long as you feel comfortable.

7. Return to your starting position and repeat on the other side.

To make it more difficult, you can raise your arms overhead, keeping them parallel with shoulders relaxed. Alternatively, you can keep your hands in front of your heart.

Heel to Toe Walk

1. Raise your arms and extend them out to the sides.

2. Place your right foot in front of your left foot, with the toe of your back foot touching the heel of your back foot.

3. Then, place your left foot in front of your right foot, with the toe of your back foot touching the heel of your back foot.

4. Continue for 20 steps.

This chapter looked at the changes that our bodies undergo throughout life and provided a brief overview of anatomy, particularly our muscles and the systems that support motion.

We also looked at the changes that occur in both muscle and bone density, leading to challenges such as osteoporosis and sarcopenia that can affect mobility and balance. We also looked at common health issues associated with aging, all of which can be managed with regular exercise.

Finally, I have provided advice on exercises for improving balance and stability. These exercises can be tailored to individual needs and progressively made more challenging to accommodate varying levels of fitness.

Key Takeaways

- Our bodies continuously change throughout life, necessitating an understanding of anatomy for better health.

- Age-related changes can lead to conditions like osteoporosis and sarcopenia, which affect muscle and bone strength.

- Balance and stability are crucial for maintaining independence in daily activities as we age.

- Regular exercise can help reduce the risks of common health issues associated with aging, improving quality of life.

Chapter 2:

Ready, Set, Go!

Before we go any further on our journey, I want you to make sure that you have gotten the green light from your doctor before starting or resuming your exercise regime. Please talk to your healthcare team if you have any health concerns.

If you have any chronic health conditions, these should not stop you from strength training, but it is wise to first consult with a professional.

Below is a Physical Activity Readiness Questionnaire known as the PAR-Q. Take this test before chatting to your doctor.

PAR-Q

Has your doctor ever said that you have a heart condition and that you should only do physical activity recommended by a doctor?

1. Do you feel pain in your chest when you do physical activity?

2. In the past month, have you had chest pain when you were not doing physical activity?

3. Do you lose your balance because of dizziness, or do you ever lose consciousness?

4. Do you have a bone or joint problem that could be made worse by a change in your physical activity?

5. Is your doctor currently prescribing drugs (for example, water pills) for your blood pressure or heart condition?

6. Do you know of any other reasons you should not do physical activity?

If you answered **YES** to any of these questions:

Talk with your doctor by phone or in person BEFORE you start becoming much more physically active or BEFORE you have a fitness appraisal. Tell your doctor about the PAR-Q and which questions you answered YES.

You may be able to do any activity you want—as long as you start slowly and build up gradually. Or, you may need to restrict your activities to those which are safe for you.

Talk with your doctor about the kinds of physical activities you wish to participate in and follow his/her advice.

Find out which community programs are safe and helpful for you.

If you answer **NO** to all of these questions:

You can start becoming more physically active—begin slowly and build up gradually. This is the safest and easiest way to go.

You can also take part in a fitness appraisal—this is an excellent way to determine your basic fitness so that you can plan the best way for you to live actively.

You should DELAY become more active if you are:

- Not feeling well because of a temporary illness such as a cold or fever—wait until you feel better.

or

- If you may be pregnant or are pregnant, talk to your doctor before you start becoming more active (Pegg, 2011).

If your health changes so that you then answer YES to any of the above questions, tell your fitness or health professional. Ask whether you should change your physical activity plan (Pegg, 2011).

Once you have filled out your PAR-Q form and are cleared to exercise, you should find out how fit and strong you are now and have a baseline idea of your health levels. You will remeasure this at the 3-, 6-, 9-, and 12-year mark and track your improvements.

How Fit and Strong Are You Now?

Mobility and Daily Activities

Rarely (1 Point) Sometimes (2 Points) Usually (3 Points) Always (4 Points)

Mobility and Daily Activities	Start	3 months	6 months	9 months	12 months
I find it easy to walk up or down two or more flights of stairs.					
I can easily lift a gallon of milk (8 lb)					
I have no trouble reaching into high cupboards or reaching down to pick up something from the					

floor				
I have no trouble taking out the trash				
I do not have trouble doing outdoor work, such as mowing the lawn, raking leaves, or gardening.				
I can easily walk a mile				
I do housework such as vacuuming and dusting on my own without difficulty				
Total:				

Mood, Energy, and Mental Health

Rarely (1 Point) Sometimes (2 Points) Usually (3 Points) Always (4 Points)

Mood, Energy, and Mental Health	Start	3 months	6 months	9 months	12 months
I feel independent					
I feel younger than my age					
I feel energetic					
I have no trouble taking out the trash					
I live an active life					
I feel strong					
I feel healthy					
I am as active as other people my age					
Total from this page:					
Total from the previous					

page:			
Total:			

Your Score

15—29 points: Your fitness level is low, and there is a lot of room for improvement in mobility, ability to complete daily tasks, and mood and mental health.

30—39 points: Your fitness level is low-to-moderate, with room for improvement in most of the above areas.

40—49 points: Your fitness level is moderate, with room for improvement in some of the above areas.

50+ points: You have an advanced fitness level; regular training will improve and maintain fitness.

Regular exercise is great for physical health, but with any physical activity, there is the chance of injury when we weigh up the risk versus the reward, it is clear that the reward far outweighs the risks. To make sure you remain safe when exercising, I have put together some tips below.

Exercise Safety

Listen to Your Body

Your body will let you know when it is tired, uncomfortable, and in pain, and if you ignore these, you are more likely to get injured. Take care of your body by:

- Getting clearance from your doctor and going for a full medical check-up before starting your fitness journey.

- Varying your exercise routine by cross-training which helps reduce the risk of overtraining.

- Creating a progressive exercise program.

- Respecting your fitness levels and meeting yourself where you are. This means beginning an exercise program that you can maintain by starting at a manageable pace.

- Increasing your duration and intensity gradually.

- Ensuring that you have at least one recovery day a week, two are ideal.

- Ensuring you rest if you are injured.

If you are sick and injured, you should take it easy. When you are ill or rehabilitating an injury, your body needs to focus on recovery. Your immune system will be working extra hard to heal you, so you should not add more stress by exercising.

When you resume exercising again, gently ease back into it, take into account the time that you have taken off, and avoid high-intensity exercise until your body is ready for it again.

When to Stop Exercising

You should stop exercising immediately if you experience any of the following.

- breathlessness

- chest pain, including pain in your neck and jaw pain that travels down your arm or pain between your shoulder blades

- a rapid or irregular heartbeat while exercising

- discomfort or pain

- joint pain that lasts more than three days of rest

Goal-Setting: Your Personal Everest

We are about to make a huge change to our lifestyles, and with any kind of change, there may be some pushback and challenges that we encounter. To make this journey easier, I suggest that we take a step-by-step approach to it.

As you begin this lifestyle change, you will go through different stages: getting motivated, starting your journey, adopting your program, and staying on track.

Getting Motivated

You are obviously curious about fitness and want to start getting healthier. Now is the time to start thinking about your goals and figuring out what you want to get out of your fitness program. You will also use this time to start thinking about any obstacles and challenges that may get in your way as you try to reach your goals. We will delve into more detail about this as we get further along in this chapter.

Starting Your Journey

Once you have gotten your goals aligned, you are ready to get started. This could mean getting your workout gear, allocating space for your home gym, and purchasing gym equipment. You will also begin to schedule time during your week to fit in your fitness sessions based on your goals.

Adopting Your Program

This is where the fun starts, as it is during this stage that you are introduced to your new program and begin learning new exercises and practicing them weekly. You will also begin to see and feel the results of your hard work, whether it is feeling fitter or your clothes beginning to fit better. This stage will last as long as you continue with your exercise program, which we hope will be forever!

Staying on Track

After six months of consistency, you will move into the maintenance stage. The good news is that this is where your fitness regime has become a part of your lifestyle. It has become your new normal, and it is harder to imagine you not exercising. You may be reaping the rewards by taking on new hobbies and even taking on more fitness and health-related activities.

Setting Realistic and Achievable Goals

Ultimately, your goal is your "why." I want you to start by asking yourself why you want to start exercising, and then I want you to continue to question yourself by asking why until you find the root of your goal.

For example:

"My goal is to lose weight."

"Why do you want to lose weight?"

"Because I am slightly overweight, and it is not healthy."

"Why is that important to you?"

"Because my family has a history of diabetes, and I want to reduce my risk of getting it."

You see, what started as a general goal that may have seemed superficial initially is actually one that is deeply rooted in health. This root goal also provides motivation when times get hard and you may find your exercise routine challenging. This is your intrinsic motivation.

Now that you have a greater goal, we are going to look at how you can create a plan so that you are successful. We will be using the SMART method:

- specific
- measurable
- attainable
- relevant
- time-based

Let's use the above goal as an example.

"My goal is to lose weight, so I reduce my risk of developing diabetes." This is your long-term goal. The first step is to break this up into smaller, manageable goals. An example of specific and short-term goals could be:

- Exercising at least 3 times a week for 30 minutes a session.

This goal is also measurable, as you can schedule these sessions in your diary and then tick them off each week.

Exercising three times a week is attainable as it gently eases you into a workout routine and allows your body to adapt and recover. As you develop the habit further and get more proficient at your movements, you can increase this to an hour each session or add an additional workout day.

This goal is relevant as it directly impacts your long-term goal and helps you achieve it.

It is time-based, as you can set this as your goal for one month, and once you have been successful at working out three times a week for a month, you can increase this.

The goals and timeframe are entirely up to you. What matters the most is that you set a goal that is truly important to you, as this will leave you with a strong desire to achieve it.

And remember, once you have reached your goals, you should celebrate your success. This can be as elaborate or simple as you want, but I usually always relate it to my fitness goals. For instance, I will reward myself with some new workout gear or gym equipment. You could pamper yourself with a massage, hike, or even a meal at your favorite restaurant. Not only do you deserve recognition for your success, but the reward also acts as motivation, pushing you to continue towards your end goal.

Eliminating Obstacles

While you think about your goals and how you are going to reach them, you should also think about obstacles and setbacks you may face. There are more common barriers, such as:

- time
- fatigue
- age or fitness levels
- health concerns

Time is the most common issue when it comes to exercising. I suggest that you make an appointment with yourself and mark that time out in your diary. You can schedule your sessions during your lunchtime break or replace your daily hour of television with an exercise session.

Fatigue is also a common reason why most people have difficulty committing to an exercise routine. The thing is, exercise gives you more energy, so once you take the first step and start exercising, you will become more energized and less fatigued.

Another misconception is that you are too old or too unfit to start working out. This is completely false. It is never too late to start, and no matter your fitness level, there is an activity that can be adapted to your needs. If you start slowly, listen to your body, and follow all safety precautions, you can successfully start an exercise regime.

If you have health concerns, you should always talk to your healthcare provider before embarking on a new exercise regime. In most cases, exercise will be approved and encouraged by your doctor, as the benefits for chronic conditions are well-researched and documented.

Home Gym Hacks: Essentials Without the Fuss

A home gym has many benefits that range from convenience to cost. You do not need to commute anywhere, and you do not need to pay any gym fees. Although the initial setup of your home gym can be expensive, in reality, you do not need any fancy equipment or special technology and there are many ways that you can set up a home gym on a budget.

Create a Budget

First, begin by listing all the gym equipment you have, such as yoga mats or a skipping rope. You can do this in an Excel spreadsheet. In your second column, list the items that you would like to purchase and prioritize them. This is your go-to list when kitting out your home gym.

Use this list to determine your budget, search for costs online for all the things you need, and get an idea of how much your home gym will cost. Do not forget to factor in shipping fees and other hidden costs.

Invest in Multitasking Equipment First

Your first purchases should be things that you can use in multiple ways, for example, dumbbells or kettlebells. These are versatile and can be used in various ways for many exercises.

Buy Second-Hand Equipment

Second-hand equipment is usually reliable, in good condition, and affordable. You can approach gyms that may be closing down or look on Facebook Marketplace.

Create a Dedicated Workout Space

This depends on how much space you have in your house that can be dedicated to your workout area. If you are fortunate enough, you can dedicate a whole room to your gym, but if not, a small corner on a balcony or in your lounge works just as well.

In order to keep your sessions safe, there are some things you should take into consideration.

Be Aware of Your Surroundings

Make sure that your area is clear of any unnecessary equipment, pets, or other things that could get in your way.

Tidy Up Afterwards

The last thing you may want to do is clean up after a hard workout, but clearing your space will ensure that you are ready for your next session without having to worry about setting things up for it. This creates convenience and safety because you will not have all your equipment lying around.

Wiping down your equipment after using it also keeps it sanitized and kills any germs or bacteria.

Invest in Adequate Storage

If you do not have a lot of space to work with, invest in storage options that can provide you with more room to move in your workout area. These can be shelves, hooks, or simple storage bins that can house your equipment so that it is out of the way.

Limit Distractions

Getting distracted can affect your concentration, and when you are working out, you want to make sure that you are focused so that you remain safe. When you have committed to your workout, make sure that you can focus and concentrate on what you are doing, and you will be less likely to experience an accident or injury.

Do Not Workout Alone

I suggest working out with a buddy to not only keep you accountable but also to provide help if anything should go wrong, such as an accident or injury.

Key Takeaways

- Always consult a healthcare provider before starting a new exercise regime.
- Use the PAR-Q to assess your readiness for increased physical activity.
- Establish a baseline fitness level to track improvements over time.
- Set realistic, achievable goals using the SMART criteria.

- Create a budget-friendly home gym with versatile equipment.

- Maintain a safe, organized workout environment to prevent injuries.

- Working out with a buddy can enhance accountability and safety.

Chapter 3:

Warm-up Wonders

In this chapter, we will explore why it is important to warm-up when it comes to getting our bodies prepared for exercise, as well as the different warm-up exercises you can use to create a great warm-up routine.

The Warm-up Wizardry

The Science Behind Warming Up

A warm-up is an activity that is performed at a slow speed and intensity, and it is done before you work. The intent behind it is to increase your body temperature, activate your neuromuscular system, and generally get your body ready to exercise (Afonso et al., 2023).

Along with physical preparedness, the warm-up also allows you to mentally get yourself ready for exercise.

When you warm-up, blood begins to pump around your body, warming up your heart and blood vessels, also known as your cardiovascular system. Blood flow to your muscles increases, and as a result, your body temperature rises. A good warm-up not only prevents injury but also aids in recovery.

You will begin your warm-up right before you are about to begin your workout routine. You will begin with an aerobic activity, and then your focus will be on the larger muscles first before moving on to the more specific muscle groups.

A warm-up does not need to be long and anything between 5-10 minutes is sufficient.

Easy Peasy Warm-up Moves

Gentle Aerobic Warm-Ups

Aerobic warm-ups are exercises that raise your heart rate and increase your breathing. Some great cardio-based warm-ups are:

- walking
- jogging
- rowing
- skipping
- cycling
- running on the spot
- jumping jacks

This should be the first movement you do when you start your warmup and should be 2 to 4 minutes long.

Gentle Warm-up Exercises

High Stepping

1. Start by standing tall. Your feet should be about shoulder-width apart. Keep your shoulder relaxed, back and down, with your arms by your side.

2. Step forward with your right leg and raise your left knee towards your chest. You can use a wall or counter for balance if you need to.

3. Using both hands or your free hand, pull your knee up close to your chest.

4. Hold for a breath and then lower the leg.

5. Repeat on the other side.

6. Alternate for the stipulated amount of repetitions or a specific amount of time.

Marching on the Spot

1. Start by standing up tall, and your feet should be underneath your hips. Keep your shoulder relaxed, back and down, with your arms by your side.

2. Begin marching by lifting your right knee up towards your waist. Try to keep your knee in line with your hip.

3. As you lift your knee, swing your left arm forward and your right arm back. This will create a marching rhythm.

4. Lower your right leg and lift your left knee while swinging your right arm forward and your left arm back.

5. Continue alternating legs and arms for 30 to 60 seconds.

Seated Hip Marches

1. Start by sitting comfortably in a chair. Your feet should be flat on the ground and underneath your hips. Keep your shoulder relaxed, back and down.

2. Hold on to the sides of the seat of your chair for balance and stability.

3. Lift your left leg with your knee bent as far as is comfortable. Place your foot down with control.

4. Repeat with the opposite leg.

5. Repeat for the stipulated amount of repetitions, alternating each leg as you do so.

Jumping Jacks

1. Start by standing up tall. Your feet should be underneath your hips. Keep your shoulder relaxed, back and down, with your arms by your side.

2. Raise your arms out to the sides and overhead and jump or step your feet out so they're slightly more than shoulder-width apart.

3. Without pausing, quickly bring your arms back down to your side and your feet together.

4. Repeat for 30 to 60 seconds.

Burpees

1. Start by standing up tall. Your feet should be underneath your hips. Keep your shoulder relaxed, back and down, with your arms by your side.

2. Gently squat down by bending your knees and lowering your body into a squat position; place your hands on the floor in front of you.

3. Walk your feet back while keeping your hands on the ground. Your body should be in a straight line from your head to your heels (this is the plank position).

4. If you are able to, carefully lower your body towards the ground by bending your elbows and doing one push-up.

5. Walk or jump your feet back toward your hands to return to the squat position.

6. Stand or jump up as you reach your hands overhead.

7. Return to the starting position.

8. Repeat for 30 to 60 seconds.

Shoulder Rolls

1. Start by standing up tall or, if you prefer, sitting down comfortably in a chair.

2. Your feet should be placed underneath your hips.

3. Gently shrug your shoulders up towards your ears.

4. Roll them back down as you squeeze your shoulder blades together.

5. Roll them towards the front and back up towards your ears.

6. Repeat for 10 rotations.

7. Roll them in the opposite direction.

Shoulder Flexions

1. Start by standing up tall or, if you prefer, sitting down comfortably in a chair.

2. Your feet should be placed underneath your hips.

3. Let your arms hang down to the side with your palms turned towards your body and thumbs facing the front.

4. Gently lift your arms up as high as you feel comfortable, pause, and then lower them back down to the sides of your body.

5. The key is to keep an upright posture throughout this exercise.

6. Repeat for the stipulated amount of repetitions.

Scapular Retraction

1. Start by standing up tall or, if you prefer, sitting down comfortably in a chair.

2. Your feet should be placed underneath your hips.

3. Place your hands on your hips, and as you do so, bring your shoulders forward, which will make your upper back round.

4. Bring your shoulders back and down while pulling your elbows back and squeezing your shoulder blades together.

5. The key here is to keep your shoulders down throughout this exercise.

6. Repeat for the stipulated amount of repetitions.

Neck Flexions

1. Start by standing up tall or, if you prefer, sitting down comfortably in a chair.

2. Your feet should be placed underneath your hips.

3. The movement starts at your neck as you imagine there is a long line from the top of your head to the bottom of your spine. Gently tuck your chin in towards your chest.

4. If you want a deeper stretch, you can place your hands behind your head and apply gentle pressure.

5. Hold this stretch for 30 to 60 seconds as you focus on relaxing your neck.

6. Lift your chin and look straight ahead, returning to your starting position.

Neck Side Flexions

1. Start by standing up tall or, if you prefer, sitting down comfortably.

2. Your feet should be placed underneath your hips.

3. Bring your left ear to your left shoulder, as far as you feel comfortable.

4. Try not to lift your shoulder to your ear.

5. Hold this stretch for 30 to 60 seconds as you focus on relaxing your neck.

6. Repeat on the other side.

Neck Rotations

1. Start by standing up tall or, if you prefer, sitting down comfortably in it.

2. Your feet should be placed underneath your hips.

3. Slowly look over your shoulder to the side.

4. Pause for a breath and return to the center.

5. Slowly look over your other shoulder.

6. Pause for a breath and return to the center.

7. Repeat for the stipulated amount of repetitions.

Hip Circles

1. Start by standing up tall, and your feet should be underneath your hips. Keep your shoulder relaxed, back and down, with your arms by your side.

2. Place your hands on your hips.

3. Gently rotate your hips in a clockwise direction. Start with small circles, and as you progress through your repetitions, expand them.

4. Rotate for 12 to 15 repetitions.

5. Return to the center and repeat in an anticlockwise direction.

Leg Circles

1. Start by standing up tall next to a chair or counter for support. Your feet should be underneath your hips. Keep your shoulder relaxed, back and down, with your arms by your side.

2. Lift your left foot off the floor, using the chair or counter for support.

3. Gently swing your leg outwards in circles. Start with small circles, and as you progress through your repetitions, expand them.

4. Rotate for 20 repetitions.

5. Rotate in the other direction for 20 repetitions.

6. Swap legs and repeat.

Arm Circles

1. Start by standing up tall, and your feet should be underneath your hips. Keep your shoulder relaxed, back and down, with your arms by your side.

2. Raise your arms out to the side of you at shoulder height. Your palms should be facing downward.

3. Rotate your arms forward in circles. Start with small circles, and as you progress through your repetitions, expand them.

4. Rotate for 20 repetitions.

5. Rotate in the other direction for 20 repetitions.

Arm Swings

1. Start by standing up tall, and your feet should be underneath your hips. Keep your shoulder relaxed, back and down, with your arms by your side.

2. Raise your arms out to the side of you at shoulder height. Your palms should be facing downward.

3. Keeping your arms straight, swing both arms towards each other until they cross in front of your chest.

4. Swing them out to your side again. Repeat this, alternating between which arm is on top of the other during crossover.

5. Repeat for 20 repetitions.

Bent Arm Shoulder Rotations

1. Start by standing up tall or, if you prefer, sitting down comfortably in it.

2. Your feet should be placed underneath your hips.

3. Raise your arms out to the sides, just below shoulder height.

4. Bend your elbows as if trying to put your fingertips on your shoulders.

5. Begin making small circles in the air with the tips of your bent elbows.

6. Repeat for 10 rotations.

7. Roll them in the opposite direction.

Wall Angels

1. Start by positioning yourself with your back against a wall with your heels about 6 inches away. You should be standing up tall, and your feet should be underneath your hips.

2. Press your lower back, upper back, and head against the wall. Keep your feet flat on the floor.

3. Raise your arms to your side, bending at a 90-degree angle, with your elbows at shoulder height and your fingers pointed upward. Your upper arms should be against the wall.

4. Slowly slide your arms upward along the wall, keeping contact with the wall throughout the movement. Your arms should straightened fully by the time your hands reach above your head.

5. Lower your arms by reversing the movement. Lower your arms back down to the starting position, keeping your elbows and wrists in contact with the wall as you do so.

6. Repeat for the stipulated amount of repetitions.

Plank Walk Outs

1. Start by standing tall. Your feet should be about shoulder-width apart. Keep your shoulder relaxed, back and down, with your arms by your side.

2. Gently bend down until your hands touch the flow.

3. Carefully and slowly walk your hands forward until you get into a plank position or as far as comfortable.

4. Pause for a second, then walk your hands back toward your feet.

5. Return to standing.

6. Continue for 30 to 60 seconds.

Bird Dogs

1. Begin by getting on your hands and knees on the floor. Use a yoga mat to keep you comfortable. Place your hands directly under your shoulders and your knees under your hips.

2. Activate your abdominal muscles to stabilize your torso and keep your back flat and your spine in a neutral position.

3. Slowly reach your right arm forward, extending it straight in front of you at shoulder height. At the same time, extend your left leg straight back, keeping it in line with your body and parallel to the floor.

4. Pause for a breath, focusing on your balance.

5. Return to your starting position by lowering your right arm and left leg back to the floor so that you are on all fours again.

6. Repeat the movement by extending your left arm forward and right leg back, following the same process.

7. Continue to alternate between sides for the stipulated amount of repetitions.

Sit to Stands

1. Begin by sitting upright on a chair with your shoulders relaxed, back and down. Keep your feet flat on the floor. Your hands can be on your lap.

2. Keep your chest up and your back straight; raise up to a standing position.

3. Lower yourself back down to your seated position.

4. Repeat for the stipulated amount of repetitions.

Quick and Easy Warm-up Routine

Here are three quick warm-up routines to get you started. You can use this as a template and create your own once you are familiar and comfortable with the exercises.

Upper Body Warm-up

Cardio

3 rounds of 30 seconds of skipping and one minute of rest between rounds.

Warm-up

1. Start by standing up tall, and your feet should be underneath your hips. Keep your shoulder relaxed, back and down, with your arms by your side.

2. Raise your arms out to the side of you at shoulder height. Your palms should be facing downward.

3. Rotate your arms forward in circles. Start with small circles, and as you progress through your repetitions, expand them.

4. Rotate for 20 repetitions.

5. Rotate in the other direction for 20 repetitions.

6. Return to your neutral standing position.

7. Gently shrug your shoulders up towards your ears.

8. Roll them back down as you squeeze your shoulder blades together.

9. Roll them towards the front and back up towards your ears.

10. Repeat for 10 rotations.

11. Roll them in the opposite direction.

12. Return to your neutral standing position.

13. The movement starts at your neck. As you imagine, there is a long line from the top of your head to the bottom of your spine. Gently tuck your chin in towards your chest.

14. If you want a deeper stretch, you can place your hands behind your head and apply gentle pressure.

15. Hold this stretch for 30 to 60 seconds as you focus on relaxing your neck.

16. Lift your chin and look straight ahead, returning to your starting position.

17. Repeat once more.

18. Return to your neutral standing position.

19. Raise your arms out to the side of you at shoulder height. Your palms should be facing downward.

20. Keeping your arms straight, swing both arms towards each other until they cross in front of your chest.

21. Swing them out to your side again. Repeat this, alternating between which arm is on top of the other during crossover.

22. Repeat for 20 repetitions.

23. Bring your left ear to your left shoulder, as far as you feel comfortable.

24. Try not to lift your shoulder to your ear.

25. Hold this stretch for 30 to 60 seconds as you focus on relaxing your neck.

26. Repeat on the other side.

27. Repeat once more.

Lower Body Warm-up

Cardio

1. Start by standing up tall, and your feet should be underneath your hips. Keep your shoulder relaxed, back and down, with your arms by your side.

2. Raise your arms out to the sides and overhead and jump or step your feet out so they're slightly more than shoulder-width apart.

3. Without pausing, quickly bring your arms back down to your side and your feet together.

4. Repeat for 30 seconds.

5. Rest for 1 minute and repeat twice more.

Warm-up

1. Start by standing tall. Your feet should be about shoulder-width apart. Keep your shoulder relaxed, back and down, with your arms by your side.

2. Step forward with your right leg and raise your left knee towards your chest. You can use a wall or counter for balance if you need to.

3. Using both hands or your free hand, pull your knee up close to your chest.

4. Hold for a breath and then lower the leg.

5. Repeat on the other side.

6. Alternate for a total of 12 repetitions

7. Return to your standing neutral position.

8. Lift your left foot off the floor, using the chair or counter for support.

9. Gently swing your leg outwards in circles. Start with small circles, and as you progress through your repetitions, expand them.

10. Rotate for 20 repetitions.

11. Rotate in the other direction for 20 repetitions.

12. Swap legs and repeat.

13. Place your hands on your hips.

14. Gently rotate your hips in a clockwise direction. Start with small circles, and as you progress through your repetitions, expand them.

15. Rotate for 12 to 15 repetitions.

16. Return to the center and repeat in an anticlockwise direction.

17. Sit down on a chair with your shoulders relaxed, back and down. Keep your feet flat on the floor. Your hands can be on your lap.

18. Keep your chest up and your back straight; raise up to a standing position.

19. Lower yourself back down to your seated position.

20. Repeat for 15 repetitions.

Full Body Warm-up

Cardio

1. Start by standing up tall, and your feet should be underneath your hips. Keep your shoulder relaxed, back and down, with your arms by your side.

2. Gently squat down by bending your knees and lowering your body into a squat position; place your hands on the floor in front of you.

3. Walk your feet back while keeping your hands on the ground. Your body should be in a straight line from your head to your heels (this is the plank position).

4. If you are able to, carefully lower your body towards the ground by bending your elbows and doing one push-up.

5. Walk or jump your feet back toward your hands to return to the squat position.

6. Stand or jump up as you reach your hands overhead.

7. Return to the starting position.

8. Repeat for 30 seconds.

9. Rest for 90 seconds and repeat twice.

Warm-up

1. Start by standing up tall, and your feet should be underneath your hips. Keep your shoulder relaxed, back and down, with your arms by your side.

2. Raise your arms out to the side of you at shoulder height. Your palms should be facing downward.

3. Keeping your arms straight, swing both arms towards each other until they cross in front of your chest.

4. Swing them out to your side again. Repeat this, alternating between which arm is on top of the other during crossover.

5. Repeat for 20 repetitions.

6. Return to a neutral standing position.

7. Lift your left foot off the floor, using the chair or counter for support.

8. Gently swing your leg outwards in circles. Start with small circles, and as you progress through your repetitions, expand them.

9. Rotate for 20 repetitions.

10. Rotate in the other direction for 20 repetitions.

11. Swap legs and repeat.

12. Position yourself with your back against a wall with your heels about 6 inches away. You should be standing up tall, and your feet should be underneath your hips.

13. Press your lower back, upper back, and head against the wall. Keep your feet flat on the floor.

14. Raise your arms to your side, bending at a 90-degree angle, with your elbows at shoulder height and your fingers pointed upward. Your upper arms should be against the wall.

15. Slowly slide your arms upward along the wall, keeping contact with the wall throughout the movement. Your arms should straightened fully by the time your hands reach above your head.

16. Lower your arms by reversing the movement. Lower your arms back down to the starting position, keeping your elbows and wrists in contact with the wall as you do so.

17. Repeat for 12 repetitions.

18. Get on your hands and knees on the floor, and use a yoga mat to keep you comfortable. Place your hands directly under your shoulders and your knees under your hips.

19. Activate your abdominal muscles to stabilize your torso and keep your back flat and your spine in a neutral position.

20. Slowly reach your right arm forward, extending it straight in front of you at shoulder height. At the same time, extend your

left leg straight back, keeping it in line with your body and parallel to the floor.

21. Pause for a breath, focusing on your balance.

22. Return to your starting position by lowering your right arm and left leg back to the floor so that you are on all fours again.

23. Repeat the movement by extending your left arm forward and right leg back, following the same process.

24. Continue to alternate between sides for 20 repetitions.

Chapter 4:

Pump It Up—Strength Training

This is where the fun begins! The next chapter is going to take you through strength training, from why it is important to the different exercises you can do. We are going to explore this form of exercise, which is often overlooked as we get older.

We are often told that we need to be careful as we get older when it comes to strength training, but this is a myth. We need to be lifting heavy (relative to ourselves) in order to stay strong and healthy. Remember that this can also mean just doing bodyweight exercises and not necessarily anything weighted; any resistance training is beneficial.

Getting started is easy, and it does not have to be complicated. It can be as simple as incorporating basic exercises into your routine. One way to start is by using your body weight for exercises like push-ups, squats, and planks. You do not need any equipment for these exercises and can be done in the comfort of your home. In this chapter, I will provide you with simple bodyweight exercises as well as options for you to use weight to make them more challenging. I will also provide you with seated versions for those of you that need modification.

As you progress, you can gradually add or increase weight or change your routine to keep it challenging and exciting. This will also help you to stay motivated and excited without it being boring.

Resistance or strength training is one of the best ways to fight the symptoms of aging. We touched on the ways that aging affects our bodies, along with some of the most common ailments that occur during old age in Chapter One, and all of those can be improved with strength training.

Strength training builds and preserves muscle, which keeps us strong, healthy, and independent, and this is for both women and men alike, regardless of age. Let's look at some of the benefits of strength training.

- Helps manage age-related muscle loss and sarcopenia.
- Fights obesity and improves metabolism.
- Reduces the risk of falls and supports functional independence.
- Improves overall quality of life.
- Improves osteoarthritis and bone health.
- Can improve your cardiovascular health.
- Improves cognitive function.
- Improves mental health.
- Reduces mortality risk.
- Improves sleep quality (Run Repeat, 2017).

The Impact of Strength Training on Cognitive Function

Strength training is not just about building muscles; it also plays an important role in improving cognitive function and improving your mental well-being. It is common for most people to believe that strength training is solely physical, but it has far-reaching effects on our mental health. Engaging in resistance exercises, such as lifting weights or using resistance bands, can stimulate various processes in the brain, positively affecting your overall cognitive abilities.

The Connection Between Exercise and Mental Health

Regular physical activity, particularly strength training, has been linked to improved mood and mental health. When we engage in exercise, our bodies release hormones that are known as endorphins. These are often referred to as the "feel-good hormones." They help to improve your mood, make you happy and can alleviate feelings of stress or sadness. This means that these endorphins are a natural and free mood booster.

In addition to endorphins, physical activity improves blood circulation. Improved blood flow means that more oxygen and nutrients reach our brain. This increase in oxygen delivery helps support brain function and cognitive performance. When we train our bodies, we are also training our minds to operate more efficiently, making our thinking clearer and sharper.

Research Supporting Exercise as a Mental Health Intervention

Numerous studies have shown that exercise can be as effective as medication in managing symptoms of depression and anxiety. One notable source is research published in the *British Journal of Sports Medicine*, which highlights the positive effects of physical activity on mental health. The findings indicate that regular exercise can significantly reduce depressive symptoms, making it an essential intervention for individuals across various age groups (British Journal of Sports Medicine, 2023).

If you are looking to not only get stronger but also want to improve your mental health, then this info is for you. For example, if you are struggling with depression, you may find that starting a simple strength training routine can improve your mood. With consistency, you might start to feel more energized and less weighed down by negative emotions.

By incorporating strength training into your routine, you are not only improving your physical health, but also looking after your mind.

Upper Body Boosters

Wall Push-Ups

1. Begin by facing a wall with your feet a little more than shoulder-width apart.

2. Position your hands by extending your arms in front of you and placing your palms flat against the wall at shoulder height. Your hands should be slightly wider than your shoulders.

3. Take a few steps back from the wall so that your body is at an angle. Your feet should be placed firmly on the ground.

4. Activate your core by tightening your abdominal muscles to support your lower back.

5. Breathe in as you bend your elbows to slowly lower your chest towards the wall. Keep your body straight and aligned from the top of your head to your feet.

6. Exhale as you straighten your arms to push your body back to the starting position.

7. Repeat for the stipulated amount of repetitions.

Chair Push-Ups

This is a slightly more challenging version of the wall push-up.

1. Start by standing up tall next to a chair and placing both hands on the backrest. Your feet should be underneath your hips. Make sure your chair is stable and will not slide.

2. Bend forward from your hips while keeping your back straight and your abdominal muscles activated.

3. Keep a slight bend in your knees you bend your elbows and bring your chest towards the chair.

4. Now straighten your arms, bringing your chest away from the chair, and repeat for the set repetitions.

You can bring your feet further away from the chair to make this exercise more challenging.

Push-Ups

This is a more challenging version of chair push-ups.

1. Begin by getting on your hands and knees on the floor. Use a yoga mat to keep you comfortable. Place your hands directly under your shoulders and your knees under your hips.

2. Walk your feet out so that you get into a plank position. Your hands should be placed slightly wider than shoulder-width apart and your feet together. Your body should form a straight line from the top of your head to your feet.

3. Activate your abdominal muscles to help you keep your body straight and engaged as you perform the movement.

4. Breathe in as you bend your elbows and lower yourself until your chest is just above the floor. Keep your hips in line with your body.

5. Press up through your palms to push your body back up to the starting positions with your arms straight and locked out.

6. Repeat for the stipulated amount of repetitions.

Bent Over Row

1. Start by standing up tall next to a chair and place one hand on the backrest. Your feet should be underneath your hips.

2. Take a step back from the chair, keep a slight bend in your knees, bend forward from your hips, and keep your back straight.

3. Place one arm by your side, keeping it straight.

4. Now, bending at the elbow, pull your arm up behind your back and return to the start position. Focus on squeezing your shoulder blades together when lifting your arm up.

5. Repeat for the stipulated amount of repetitions.

6. Swap sides and repeat on the other hand.

As you progress, you can add weights to the movement and use one dumbbell in each hand.

Seated Row

1. Start by sitting comfortably in a chair; your feet should be flat on the ground and underneath your hips. Keep your shoulder relaxed, back and down.

2. Make a fist with both of your hands and extend your arms out in front of you.

3. Pull your elbows back behind you as you squeeze your shoulder blades together at the end of the movement.

4. Remember to keep your chest up throughout this exercise.

5. Repeat for the stipulated amount of repetitions.

Bicep Curl

You can do this exercise both seated and standing.

1. Start by standing up tall or, if you prefer, sitting down comfortably in a chair.

2. Let your arms hang by your sides with your palms facing forward. Make a fist with both of your hands.

3. From this position, curl your arm from the elbow all the way up until your closed fist almost touches your shoulder, and then slowly lower it back down.

4. Repeat on the other side with the other arm.

5. Repeat for the stipulated amount of repetitions, alternating arms as you do so.

This exercise can also be done with both arms at the same time.

As you progress, you can add weights to the movement and use one dumbbell in each hand.

Shoulder Press Ups

1. You can do this exercise both seated and standing.

2. Start by standing up tall or, if you prefer, sitting down comfortably in a chair.

3. Bring your hand up to either side of your shoulders with your palms facing forward. Make a fist with both your hands.

4. Now press up and slowly lift your hands up above your head as far as you can go, and then slowly lift them back down to the start position.

5. Make sure you do not over-arch your back as you do so.

6. Repeat for the stipulated amount of repetitions.

As you progress, you can add weights to the movement and use one dumbbell in each hand.

Tricep Lifts

1. Start by sitting comfortably towards the front of your chair, and your feet should be flat on the ground and underneath your hips. Keep your shoulder relaxed, back and down.

2. Put your hands on either side of the seat of the chair near your hips or on the armrests.

3. Lean slightly forward at the hips while keeping your back straight.

4. Now press through your hands, straightening your elbows and lifting your buttocks off the chair, if you can.

5. Slowly lower your buttocks back to the chair by bending at your elbows.

6. Repeat for the stipulated amount of repetitions.

Shoulder Taps

1. Begin by getting on your hands and knees on the floor. Use a yoga mat to keep you comfortable. Place your hands directly under your shoulders and your knees under your hips.

2. Start in a high plank with your palms flat, hands shoulder-width apart, shoulders stacked directly above your wrists, but keep your knees on the floor and raise your upper body only.

3. Tap your right hand to your left shoulder while keeping your core and glutes activated and trying to keep your hips as still as possible.

4. Do the same thing with your left hand on your right shoulder. That's 1 rep.

5. Repeat the stipulated number of repetitions, alternating sides.

To make this easier, try separating your legs a little more.

Side Arm Raises

1. Start by standing tall. Your feet should be about shoulder-width apart. Keep your shoulders relaxed, back and down, with your arms by your side.

2. Your palms should be turned towards your thighs; make a fist with both of them.

3. Keeping your arms straight, raise both arms to the side to shoulder level and control them as you lower them back down.

4. Repeat for the stipulated amount of repetitions.

You can add weights to the movement as you progress and use one dumbbell in each hand.

Front Arm Raises

1. Start by standing tall. Your feet should be about shoulder-width apart. Keep your shoulders relaxed, back and down, with your arms by your side.

2. Your palms should be turned backward; make a fist with both of them.

3. Keeping your arms straight, raise both arms to the front to shoulder level and control them as you lower them back down.

4. Repeat for the stipulated amount of repetitions.

You can add weights to the movement as you progress and use one dumbbell in each hand.

Lower Body Lifters

Partial/Half Squat

1. Start by standing up tall next to a chair or counter if you need support. Keep your shoulders relaxed, back and down.

2. Your feet should be shoulder-width apart, with your toes either facing forward or slightly outwards.

3. You can hold on to the chair for support or raise your arms in front of you.

4. Activate your midline carefully, bend your hips, and sit back as you would if you were to sit on a chair.

5. As you sit back, keep your chest up and your core tight, and go no lower than 45 degrees.

6. As you stand back up, put equal weight through both legs, ensuring your feet stay flat on the floor throughout.

7. Make sure your knees stay in the line of your toes, they don't go forward past your toes, and they aren't moving inward throughout the exercise.

8. Repeat for the stipulated amount of repetitions.

Chair Knee Extensions

1. Start by sitting comfortably in a chair; your feet should be flat on the ground and underneath your hips. Keep your shoulder relaxed, back and down.

2. Life up one of your legs, extending at the knee.

3. Pause and hold this position for a breath at the top of the movement, squeezing the muscles at the front of the thigh before lowering your leg back down.

4. Keep your movements controlled and slow.

5. Lower your leg, swap sides, and repeat.

6. Alternate legs and repeat for the set repetitions.

Chair Knee Flexion

1. Start by sitting comfortably in a chair; your feet should be flat on the ground and underneath your hips. Keep your shoulder relaxed, back and down. Move towards the front of your seat.

2. Bring your left foot back towards your chair as far as it can go.

3. Return to the start position and repeat with your right foot.

4. Alternate legs and repeat for the set amount of repetitions.

Heel Slides

1. Start by sitting comfortably in a chair; your feet should be flat on the ground and underneath your hips. Keep your shoulder relaxed, back and down. Move towards the front of your seat.

2. Keep your abdominal muscles engaged and tight. Keep your chest raised.

3. Put both of your hands at the sides of your chair and grip the seat to keep it stable.

4. Extend one leg far out in front of your body and point your toes forward. The extended leg's foot should be diagonal to the hips. If using a blanket or other item, place your foot on top. The other leg should be naturally bent, close to the body, with the foot planted on the floor.

5. Using your extended leg, keep your foot flat and push against the floor, then drag your foot slowly toward your body until it reaches the flexed position of the other leg.

6. While keeping pressure, extend the leg back to the starting position.

7. A single rep is when performing the full movement of pulling and then pushing the foot back to the starting position.

8. Alternate legs and repeat for the set amount of repetitions.

Squat

1. Start by standing up tall next to a chair or counter if you need support. Keep your shoulders relaxed, back and down.

2. Your feet should be shoulder-width apart, with your toes either facing forward or slightly outwards.

3. You can hold on to the chair for support or raise your arms in front of you.

4. Activate your midline carefully, bend your hips, and sit back as you would if you were to sit on a chair.

5. As you sit back, keep your chest up and your core tight; aim to go to 90 degrees or slightly lower.

6. As you stand back up, put equal weight through both legs, ensuring your feet stay flat on the floor throughout.

7. Make sure your knees stay in the line of your toes; they don't go forward past your toes, and they aren't moving inward throughout the exercise.

8. Repeat for the stipulated amount of repetitions.

As you progress, you can add weights to the movement and use one dumbbell in each hand.

Reverse Lunge

1. Start by standing up tall next to a chair or counter if you need support. Keep your shoulders relaxed, back and down.

2. Your feet should be slightly wider than hip-width apart.

3. Take a large step backward and gently lower your back knee to the floor.

4. Keep your body upright and make sure that your front knee is not tracking over your foot. Your shin should be perpendicular to the floor.

5. Pushing up through your front foot, bring yourself back up to a standing position.

6. Swap sides and repeat on the opposite leg.

7. Repeat for the stipulated amount of repetitions alternating on each side as you do so.

Forward Lunge

1. Start by standing up tall next to a chair or counter if you need support. Keep your shoulders relaxed, back and down.

2. Your feet should be slightly wider than hip-width apart.

3. Take a large step forward and gently lower your back knee to the floor.

4. Keep your body upright and make sure that your front knee is not tracking over your foot. Your shin should be perpendicular to the floor.

5. Pushing up through your back foot, bring yourself back up to a standing position.

6. Swap sides and repeat on the opposite leg.

7. Repeat for the stipulated amount of repetitions alternating on each side as you do so.

Lateral Lunges

1. Start by standing tall. Your feet should be about hip-width apart. Keep your shoulders relaxed, back and down, with your hands on your hips or clasped in front of your chest.

2. Carefully take a wide step to your right with your right foot. Keep your left leg straight as you begin to bend your right knee.

3. As you step to the side, push your hips back and lower your body toward your right knee. Make sure that your right knee stays aligned with your right foot and does not extend past your toes.

4. Keep your back straight by keeping your chest up throughout the movement. Try to avoid rounding your back.

5. Lower your body until your right thigh is parallel to the ground or as low as you can comfortably go. Hold this position for one breath.

6. Push through your right foot to return to the starting position, and activate your glutes and leg muscles as you stand up.

7. Once you've completed your repetitions on the right side, repeat the movement on your left side by stepping to the left and bending your left knee while keeping your right leg straight.

8. Alternate sides for the desired number of repetitions.

Seated Calf Raises

1. Start by sitting comfortably in a chair; your feet should be flat on the ground and underneath your hips. Keep your shoulder relaxed, back and down. Move towards the front of your seat.

2. Bring your feet back so your heels are behind your knees.

3. From this position, lift your heels up off the floor, coming up onto your toes.

4. Hold briefly and gently lower your heels back down.

5. Repeat for the stipulated amount of repetitions

Calf Raises

1. Start by standing up tall next to a chair or counter if you need support. Keep your shoulders relaxed, back and down.

2. Your feet should be hip-width apart.

3. Keep your knees straight and hold on to the chair for support if needed.

4. Come up onto your toes and raise your heels off the floor.

5. Hold this position briefly before lowering yourself back down.

6. Repeat for the stipulated amount of repetitions

Kettlebell Deadlift

1. Start by standing tall. Your feet should be about shoulder-width apart. Keep your shoulders relaxed, back and down, with your arms by your side.

2. Place the kettlebell on the floor between your feet. You should be facing the kettlebell.

3. Bend forward at your hips and bend your knees slightly. Keep your back straight and your chest up as you lower your body toward the kettlebell.

4. Reach down and take hold of the kettlebell handle with both hands, making sure that you have a firm grip.

5. Before you lift, activate your midline and core muscles to stabilize your body.

6. Push through your heels and extend your hips and knees simultaneously to lift the kettlebell. Keep the kettlebell close to your body as you stand upright.

7. At the top of the lift, stand tall with your shoulders back and chest forward. The kettlebell should be hanging in front of your thighs.

8. To lower the kettlebell, bend your hips first, then bend your knees. Keep your back straight as you guide the kettlebell back down toward the floor.

9. Reset your position and repeat the movement for the desired number of repetitions.

Kettlebell Swings

1. Start by standing tall. Your feet should be about shoulder-width apart. Keep your shoulders relaxed, back and down, with your arms by your side. The kettlebell should be placed on the ground in front of you. Your toes should be facing outwards slightly.

2. Bend at your hips and knees as you lower your body. Your back should be flat, and your midline should be activated. Take hold of the kettlebell handle with both hands with your palms facing towards you.

3. Carefully pull the kettlebell slightly back between your legs and allow it to rest between your inner thighs. This is your starting position.

Glute Bridges

1. Begin by lying on your back on a mat or flat surface with your knees bent and feet flat on the floor, hip-width apart. Your arms should be at your sides, palms facing down.

2. Keep your feet close to your glutes so that they are within comfortable reaching distance.

3. Before lifting your hips, activate your midline and stabilize your core muscles.

4. Press through your heels and squeeze your glutes as you carefully lift your hips off the ground.

5. Keep your back straight and try not to overarch and hyperextend excessively.

6. Raise your hips until your body forms a straight line from your shoulders to your knees, and hold this position for a breath while you focus on squeezing your glutes.

7. When you are done, slowly lower your hips back down to the floor. Make sure that you control the movement as you do so.

8. Repeat for the stipulated amount of repetitions.

Step-Ups

1. Start by standing tall, facing a sturdy bench, step, or raised platform. Your feet should be about hip-width apart. Keep your shoulders relaxed, back and down, with your arms by your side.

2. Decide which leg you want to start with and step forward with that foot onto the step or platform.

3. Press down through the heel of your leading foot and push your body upward, lifting your back leg off the ground as you step up. Your knee should be aligned over your ankle.

4. At the top of the movement, stand up tall with your starting leg. Lock out your knee and bring your back leg up to the step.

5. When you have completed the step up, and you want to return to your starting position, step back down with your second leg, followed by your starting leg.

6. Control your movement as you come down.

7. Repeat the stipulated number of repetitions, alternating with each leg.

Wall Sits

1. Find a flat wall with enough space for you to comfortably stand against it. Stand about two feet away from it with your feet hip-width apart.

2. Carefully lean back against the wall, making sure that your back is flat against it.

3. Slowly slide down the wall until your thighs are parallel to the ground or as low as you can comfortably and safely go.

4. Keep your knees directly above your ankles, forming a 90 degrees angle.

5. Your feet remain hip-width apart, with the soles of your feet flat on the ground. Make sure your knees do not go past your toes.

6. Keep your midline and core tight to stabilize your body and protect your posture.

7. Hold this position for as long as required or for as long as you feel comfortable. You can increase your time as you get stronger.

8. When you are done, you can come out of the wall and sit by carefully sliding yourself back up the wall to your standing position.

Side Leg Raises

1. Begin by lying on your side on a mat or flat surface with your knees bent and feet flat on the floor, hip-width apart. You can either rest your head on your arm or place a cushion under your head to make yourself comfortable.

2. Keep your body in a straight line from your head to your feet, with your legs stacked on top of each other.

3. Bend your bottom leg at your knee while keeping it flat on the ground to keep you stable. You can also keep it straight if you prefer.

4. Keep your top leg straight as you slowly lift it up toward the ceiling. Activate your glutes and midline as you raise your leg.

5. Lift your leg till it is about 45° off the ground or as high as you feel comfortable. Hold this position for a breath while making sure your body remains in a straight line.

6. Slowly lower your leg back down to the starting position.

7. Repeat for the stipulated amount of repetitions on one side, then swap sides and repeat on the other.

Core Crusaders

Plank

1. Begin by getting on your hands and knees on the floor. Use a yoga mat to keep you comfortable. Place your hands directly under your shoulders and your knees under your hips.

2. Your hands should be placed slightly wider than shoulder-width apart and your feet together. Tuck your toes under and lift your body off the ground, creating a straight line from your head to your heels.

3. Engage your abdominal muscles, core muscles, glutes, and legs to maintain a stable position and prevent your hips from dropping.

4. Keep your head in a neutral position, looking at the floor slightly ahead of your hands. Avoid tilting your head up or dropping it down.

5. Maintain this position for the desired duration, focusing on your breathing and staying relaxed.

6. When you are ready to release the hold, gently lower your knees to the ground and return to a resting position.

Cobra

1. Begin by lying face down on the floor. Use a yoga mat to keep you comfortable. Place your hands directly under your shoulders and hands facing forward. Extend your legs and point your toes away from your body.

2. Breathe out, press your hips into the mat or floor, and push your chest upwards and away from the floor while keeping your hips on the ground. Your arms should extend fully.

3. This will arch your lower back and you will feel a stretch in the muscles of your chest and abdomen. Hold this position for 15 to 30 seconds.

4. When you are ready to release, slowly lower your chest back to the floor.

Crunch

1. Begin by lying on your back. Use a yoga mat to keep you comfortable. Bend your knees and keep your feet flat on the ground, with your heels positioned 12 to 18 inches away from you.

2. Place your hands behind your head for support. You will keep this position throughout the exercise.

3. Breathe out as you activate your midline and bring your chin slightly towards your chest. Curl your torso towards your thighs.

4. Keep your neck relaxed and keep your chin towards your chest. Your feet and lower back stay on the floor throughout the whole movement. Continue to curl yourself up until your upper back lifts off the floor.

5. Hold this position briefly.

6. Return to your starting position by gently curling back down.

7. Repeat for the stipulated amount of repetitions.

Reverse Ab Crunch

1. Begin by lying on your back. Use a yoga mat to keep you comfortable. Bend your knees and keep your feet flat on the ground, with your heels positioned 12 to 18 inches away from you.

2. Spread your arms out to your sides with your palms facing down.

3. Activate your midline by bracing your abdominal muscles and slowly lift your feet off the floor, raising your knees directly above your hips while maintaining a 90-degree bend in the knees.

4. Hold this position and breathe normally. Use your arms as a balance support.

5. Carefully lift your hips off the mat, rolling your spine up as if trying to bring your knees towards your head. You can use your arms and hands to help keep your balance as you continue to curl up until your spine cannot roll any further. Hold this position for a breath.

6. Breathe in and carefully lower your spine back towards the floor in a controlled manner, moving your upper thighs backward until they are positioned directly over your hips. Continue rolling out until your spine and hips contact the mat and your knees are positioned directly over your hips with a 90-degree bend with your lower leg.

7. Repeat for the stipulated amount of repetitions.

Side Plank

1. Begin by lying on your side with your legs extended and the left leg lying directly on the right. You can use a yoga mat to keep you comfortable.

2. Bend your right leg, but keep your left leg straight. The inside of your left foot should remain in touch with the floor.

3. Lift your torso by propping yourself up on your right arm, keeping your elbow bent at 90 degrees. It should be positioned right under your shoulder.

4. Keep your head in line with your spine, with your hips and knees still in contact with the floor.

5. Breathe out as you activate your midline to stiffen your spine and brace.

6. Gently lift your hips and right leg off the ground, keeping your head still in with your spine.

7. Hold for as long as required before carefully lowering yourself down to the ground.

8. Swap sides and repeat.

Bicycle Crunches

1. Begin by lying on your back. Use a yoga mat to keep you comfortable. Bend your knees and keep your feet flat on the ground, with your heels positioned 12 to 18 inches away from you.

2. Place your hands behind your head for support. You will keep this position throughout the exercise.

3. Carefully lift both feet off the floor, moving your knees towards your torso until your thighs align vertically to the floor, creating a 90-degree angle at your hips. Keep the 90-degree bend at the knee and relax your feet, allowing them to point away from your body.

4. Bring your right knee towards your chest in a straight line and extend your left leg while keeping it off the floor. At the same time, lift your shoulders off the floor and bring your left elbow towards your right knee.

5. Your lower back should remain pressed against the floor.

6. Do these two movements simultaneously.

7. Move carefully and slowly until your elbow touches or almost touches your opposite knee. Hold for a breath and return to the starting position.

8. Repeat on the opposite side.

9. Repeat for the stipulated amount of repetitions.

Seated Knee to Chest

1. Start by sitting comfortably towards the front of your chair; your feet should be flat on the ground and underneath your hips. Keep your shoulder relaxed, back and down.

2. Hold onto both sides of the seat of the chair for balance and to keep you stable.

3. Place both feet far out in front of your body and point your toes to the ceiling. Both of your feet should be diagonal to your hips.

4. Slowly raise both legs closer to your body while bending your knees. Try to bring your knees as close to your chest as possible.

5. Slowly perform this motion in the exact opposite direction back to the starting position. This equals one "rep".

6. Repeat for the stipulated amount of repetitions.

Seated Extended Knee Raises

1. Start by sitting comfortably towards the front of your chair; your feet should be flat on the ground and underneath your hips. Keep your shoulder relaxed, back and down.

2. Hold onto both sides of the seat of the chair for balance and to keep you stable.

3. Place both feet far out in front of your body and point your toes to the ceiling. Both of your feet should be diagonal to your hips.

4. Lift one of your legs up to the highest point possible (optimal range ending at the hips) without moving the center of your body. The other leg will stay in the starting position.

5. Slowly lower the leg back to the starting position, then repeat with the opposite leg.

6. Kicking both legs equals one "rep".

7. Repeat for the stipulated amount of repetitions.

Seated Leg Kicks

This exercise is very similar to that of the seated extended leg raises in terms of motion.

1. Start by sitting comfortably towards the front of your chair; your feet should be flat on the ground and underneath your hips. Keep your shoulder relaxed, back and down.

2. Hold onto both sides of the seat of the chair for balance and to keep you stable.

3. Place both feet far out in front of your body and point your toes to the ceiling. Both of your feet should be diagonal to your hips.

4. Lift one of your legs up to the highest point possible (optimal range ending at the hips) without moving the center of your body. The other leg will stay in the starting position.

5. Slowly lower the leg back to the starting position, then repeat with the opposite leg.

6. Pretend that you are swimming, kicking your legs in the water.

7. Kicking both legs equals one "rep".

8. Repeat for the stipulated amount of repetitions.

Seated Twists

1. Using a medicine ball or something similar, hold it in front of your body, gripping the sides of the medicine ball with your elbows bent.

2. Sit comfortably towards the front of your chair; your feet should be flat on the ground and underneath your hips. Keep your shoulder relaxed, back and down.

3. Lift your medicine ball a couple of inches off your lap, then rotate your upper body to the right, keeping the ball in front of your body.

4. Gently rotate it towards the middle of your body, then rotate to your left, and finish by rotating back to the middle.

5. Each "rep" is one full rotation.

6. Repeat for the stipulated amount of repetitions.

Full Body Fitness

Inchworm

1. Start by standing tall. Your feet should be about shoulder-width apart. Keep your shoulders relaxed, back and down, with your arms by your side.

2. Bend at your waist and reach down towards the ground, trying to keep your legs straight. If you can't touch the ground, it's okay to bend your knees slightly.

3. Place your hands on the ground in front of you and walk them forward until you are in a plank position (hands under your shoulders, body in a straight line).

4. Keep your core engaged to ensure your body stays straight and stable.

5. Take small steps to walk your feet towards your hands, keeping your legs as straight as possible. This will bring you back into a standing position.

6. Once you are back in the starting position, bend forward again and repeat the movement.

7. Repeat for the stipulated amount of repetitions.

Bear Crawl

1. Begin by getting on your hands and knees on the floor. Use a yoga mat to keep you comfortable. Place your hands directly under your shoulders and your knees under your hips.

2. Raise your knees off the ground a few inches while keeping your back flat. This is your starting bear crawl position.

3. Move your right hand and left foot forward at the same time, followed by your left hand and right foot. Aim to keep your body low and controlled.

4. As you move, keep your midline active and stabilize your body. You do not want your hips to sway.

5. Continue to alternate moving your hands and feet, crawling forward for a set distance or number of steps.

If you would like to make it more challenging, you can also crawl backward by moving your opposite limbs in the same manner.

Mountain Climbers

1. Begin in a high plank position with your hands directly under your shoulders and your body in a straight line from head to heels.

2. Engage your abdominal muscles, core muscles, glutes, and legs to maintain a stable position and prevent your hips from dropping.

3. Keep your head in a neutral position, looking at the floor slightly ahead of your hands. Avoid tilting your head up or dropping it down.

4. Quickly bring your right knee toward your chest while keeping your left leg extended.

5. As you return your right foot back to the starting position, drive your left knee toward your chest at the same time.

6. Continue alternating by quickly bringing your right and left knees toward your chest, mimicking a running motion while maintaining the plank position.

7. Aim to keep your hips down and your body in a straight line throughout the movement. Avoid lifting your hips too high.

8. Repeat for the stipulated amount of repetitions.

Renegade Row

1. Begin in a high plank position, gripping a pair of dumbbells placed on the floor, or you can just use your hands if you prefer. They should be directly under your shoulders and your body in a straight line from head to heels.

2. Place your feet slightly wider than shoulder-width apart to help maintain balance.

3. Engage your abdominal muscles, core muscles, glutes, and legs to maintain a stable position and prevent your hips from dropping.

4. Shift your weight slightly to one side and lift the dumbbell in the opposite hand off the floor, pulling it towards your rib cage while keeping your elbow close to your body.

5. Carefully lower the dumbbell back to the ground with control while maintaining your plank position.

6. Repeat on the other side and perform the same rowing motion with the opposite arm, lifting the dumbbell towards your rib cage.

7. Alternate between sides for the desired number of repetitions or duration.

Squat to Overhead Press

1. Start by standing up tall. Keep your shoulders relaxed, back and down. Hold two dumbbells at shoulder height with your palms facing forward and elbows bent.

2. Your feet should be shoulder-width apart, with your toes either facing forward or slightly outwards.

3. Lower your body into a squat by bending at your hips and sitting back as you would if you were to sit on a chair. Make sure your knees stay in the line of your toes; they don't go forward past your toes, and they aren't moving inward throughout the exercise.

4. As you sit back, keep your chest up and your core tight; aim to go to 90 degrees or slightly lower.

5. As you reach the bottom of the squat (thighs parallel to the ground or lower), transition to the overhead press position by keeping the weights at your shoulders.

6. As you stand back up, put equal weight through both legs, ensuring your feet stay flat on the floor throughout while lifting the weights overhead by extending your arms fully overhead as you stand upright, ensuring your elbows are locked at the top.

7. Lower the weights back to shoulder height as you prepare for the next squat.

8. Repeat for the stipulated amount of repetitions.

Suitcase Carry

1. Start by standing up tall. Keep your shoulders relaxed, back and down. Stand with your feet shoulder-width apart, holding a dumbbell or kettlebell in one hand at your side.

2. Activate your midline to maintain stability and posture throughout the movement.

3. Keep your shoulders back and chest up, ensuring your body is straight.

4. Begin walking forward, taking small, controlled steps while maintaining your posture and balance.

5. Keep the kettlebell or dumbbell close to your body, and avoid leaning to one side. Maintain a neutral spine and avoid hunching your shoulders.

6. Continue walking for a set distance or duration, such as 20 to 30 feet, or for a specific time, like 30 seconds to 1 minute.

7. Once you have completed your distance or time frame, switch the weight to the other hand and repeat the carry in the opposite direction.

8. Once completed, lower the weight safely to the ground.

Farmers Carry

1. Start by standing up tall. Keep your shoulders relaxed, back and down. Stand with your feet shoulder-width apart, holding a dumbbell or kettlebell in both hands at your side.

2. Activate your midline to maintain stability and posture throughout the movement.

3. Keep your shoulders back and chest up, ensuring your body is straight.

4. Begin walking forward, taking small, controlled steps while maintaining your posture and balance.

5. Keep the kettlebell or dumbbell close to your body. Maintain a neutral spine and avoid hunching your shoulders.

6. Continue walking for a set distance or duration, such as 20 to 30 feet, or for a specific time, like 30 seconds to 1 minute.

7. Once you have completed your distance or time frame, switch the weight to the other hand and repeat the carry in the opposite direction.

8. Once completed, lower the weight safely to the ground.

Key Takeaways

- Strength training is essential for maintaining health and strength as we age.

- Bodyweight exercises are a great starting point and can be modified for different fitness levels.

- Regular strength training can enhance cognitive function and improve mental health.

- Exercise releases endorphins that boost mood and alleviate stress.

- A variety of exercises targeting different muscle groups can be easily incorporated into daily routines.

Chapter 5:

Cool Down Like a Pro

You have just finished your work, and you are hot and slightly sweating. You have done your strength portion and worked your muscles. Time to take a shower and eat something to help with your recovery. Hang on a second, not just yet.

Just like warming up, cooling down is just as important to your exercise program as the workout itself.

Some reasons to cool down after a workout include:

- reducing your chances of getting delayed onset muscle soreness (DOMS)
- provides stress relief
- gradually lowering your heart rate
- decreasing your risk of injury
- improving your flexibility
- prevents blood pooling (Grant, 2022)

Reducing Delayed Onset Muscle Soreness (DOMS)

An effective cool-down will reduce the risk of delayed onset muscle soreness, commonly known as DOMS. This refers to the soreness that you may feel after a workout, especially if you are trying new exercises or increasing your workout intensity. By allowing your muscles to gradually return to their normal state, you can reduce this discomfort. A simple way to cool down could include gentle stretching and low-intensity movements. For instance, if you just finished a run, walking for five to ten minutes can help shake off the soreness and help prepare your muscles for recovery.

Providing Stress Relief

Cooling down also provides an excellent opportunity for stress relief. After you exercise, your body produces endorphins, which are also known as our feel-good hormones. When you take some time to cool down, you let your body savor this good feeling, and it allows you to relax your mind while doing so.

During your cool down, you can practice deep-breathing techniques which can provide you with further help to manage stress. For example, after your exercise, try sitting or lying down comfortably, closing your eyes, and taking deep, slow breaths. This not only helps decrease your heart rate but also calms your mind and sets a peaceful tone for the rest of your day.

Gradually Lowering Your Heart Rate

When we warm-up and exercise, we spike our heart rates, and we need to bring this down gently cooling down helps us to do that.

During intense physical activity, your heart rate increases significantly to support your body while exercising. Moving too quickly from high intensity to complete rest can give your body a bit of a shock. A good cooling-down routine helps your heart to adjust and reduces the chance of dizziness or faintness. After your workout, take three to five minutes to perform light activities, such as walking or slow cycling, followed by gentle stretches. This will help your body move from an active state to a resting state safely.

Decreasing the Risk of Injury

When your muscles are not properly supported during a workout, you are more at risk for injuries. Cooling down reduces your risk by allowing your muscles to relax and recover gradually. Good, well-thought-of cool-down stretches can improve your muscle's elasticity and joint flexibility, which makes your muscles and joints more stable. Focus on the muscle groups you worked on during your session. For instance, if you are engaged in lower body exercises, take some time to stretch your hamstrings, quadriceps, and calves. These stretches will encourage blood flow to these areas and promote healing and recovery.

Improving Flexibility

Another advantage of cooling down is that it helps improve your flexibility, and as we know, as we get older, our flexibility lessens. You may have been under the impression that stretching was only a warm-up activity, but it is equally beneficial after a workout.

After you have worked out, your muscles are still warm and, therefore, more receptive to stretching. By adding static stretches during your cool-down, you can help lengthen your muscles and improve your range of motion. Simple exercises such as reaching for your toes or doing a butterfly stretch are two simple stretches that you can do as a cooldown. The more consistent you are, the better, as this habit will help to improve your flexibility over time, making future workouts easier and more effective.

Preventing Blood Pooling

Blood can pool in your lower extremities when you stop exercising suddenly, particularly after high-intensity workouts. This can lead to feelings of lightheadedness or dizziness.

Slowing down and moving gently after exercise helps maintain circulation.

Stretch It Out: Flexibility, Fun

Neck Extension Stretch

1. Start by standing up tall or, if you prefer, sitting down comfortably in a chair.
2. Your feet should be placed underneath your hips.
3. Place your arms on your thighs, or let them hang to your side.
4. Carefully lean your head straight back, looking up to the ceiling and going as far back as you feel comfortable. Do not push into any pain.
5. Hold for 30 to 60 seconds.
6. Release and return to neutral.

Neck Flexion Stretch

1. Start by standing up tall or, if you prefer, sitting down comfortably in a chair.

2. Your feet should be placed underneath your hips.

3. Place your arms on your thighs, or let them hang to your side.

4. Bring your chin towards your chest, starting the movement from your neck. Think about creating a long line from the top of your head to the base of your spine.

5. If you would like to increase the stretch, you can place your hands on the back of your head and apply gentle pressure.

6. Hold for 30 to 60 seconds.

7. Carefully return your head to the starting position, lifting your chin and looking straight ahead.

Neck Rotation Stretch

1. Start by standing up tall or, if you prefer, sitting down comfortably in a chair.

2. Your feet should be placed underneath your hips.

3. Place your arms on your thighs, or let them hang to your side.

4. Look over to your left shoulder as far as you feel comfortable.

5. Hold for 30 to 60 seconds.

6. Look over to your right shoulder as far as you feel comfortable.

7. Hold for 30 to 60 seconds.

8. Carefully return your head to the starting position.

Levator Scapula Stretch

1. Start by standing up tall or, if you prefer, sitting down comfortably in a chair.

2. Your feet should be placed underneath your hips.

3. Place the hand on the side you are stretching behind the shoulder to stabilize your shoulder blade. If unable to do this, just perform the exercise without placing one hand behind your shoulder.

4. Carefully turn your head to about 45 degrees to one side and bring your head down as if you are looking at your knee on that side.

5. You will feel a stretch on the opposite side. You are looking behind the neck and shoulder.

6. If you would like to increase the stretch, place your hand on the back of your head and apply gentle pressure.

7. Hold for 30 to 60 seconds.

8. Carefully return your head to the starting position.

Neck Side Stretch

1. Start by standing up tall or, if you prefer, sitting down comfortably in a chair.

2. Your feet should be placed underneath your hips.

3. Bring your ear down to your shoulder; do not bring your shoulder up to your ear; leave your shoulder relaxed. Go as far as you feel comfortable.

4. To increase the stretch, place your hand on the side of your head and apply gentle pressure.

5. Hold this position for 30 to 60 seconds.

6. Repeat the stretch on each side 2 to 3 times, gradually increasing the duration and intensity as your neck becomes more flexible.

Thoracic Rotation Stretch

1. Start by standing up tall or, if you prefer, sitting down comfortably in a chair.

2. Your feet should be placed underneath your hips.

3. Cross your arms over your chest and gently rotate around until you feel a stretch in your upper back.

4. Hold this position for 30 to 60 seconds and repeat on the opposite side.

Shoulder and Arm Overhead Stretch

1. Start by standing up tall or, if you prefer, sitting down comfortably in a chair.

2. Your feet should be placed underneath your hips.

3. Interlace your fingers and turn your palms away from you.

4. Raise your arms up above your head, towards the ceiling, and push-up as far as you can.

5. Hold this position for 30 to 60 seconds.

Upper Arm and Shoulder Stretch

1. Start by standing up tall or, if you prefer, sitting down comfortably in a chair.

2. Your feet should be placed underneath your hips.

3. Place one arm straight in front of your body and use your other hand to hug the straight arm to your body.

4. Hold this position for 30 to 60 seconds.

5. Release and repeat on the other side.

Chest Stretch

1. Start by standing up tall or, if you prefer, sitting down comfortably in a chair.

2. Your feet should be placed underneath your hips.

3. Raise your arms straight up in front of you, parallel to the floor.

4. Now, bring your arms out to the side, pulling as far back as you can and squeezing your shoulder blades together while keeping your posture upright.

5. If you have difficulty holding your arms at 90 degrees (or parallel to the floor), you can hold your arms lower (45 degrees).

6. Hold this position for 30 to 60 seconds.

Hamstring Stretch

1. Start by standing up tall next to a chair or counter for support. Your feet should be underneath your hips. Keep your shoulder relaxed, back and down, with your arms by your side.

2. Place one foot out in front of you while keeping your knees straight and keeping your heels on the floor at all times.

3. Slightly bend your back knee and keep your toes facing forward.

4. Keeping your hips square and your back straight, lean forward, feeling the stretch in the back of your leg.

5. Hold this position for 30 to 60 seconds and then change legs.

Calf Stretch

1. Start by standing up tall next to a chair or counter for support. Your feet should be underneath your hips. Keep your shoulder relaxed, back and down, with your arms by your side.

2. Place one foot behind you, making sure your toes are facing forward throughout the exercise.

3. Now, bring your front knee towards the chair, ensuring that your heels remain in contact with the floor at all times.

4. Hold this position for 30 to 60 seconds and then change legs.

Groin Stretch

1. Start by standing up tall next to a chair or counter for support. Your feet should be underneath your hips. Keep your shoulder relaxed, back and down, with your arms by your side.

2. Take one large step out to the side and face your toes outwards.

3. Shift your weight to one side, bending that knee. You will feel a stretch on the inner thigh of the straight leg.

4. Hold this position for 30 to 60 seconds and then change legs.

Quad Stretch

1. Start by standing up tall next to a chair or counter for support. Your feet should be underneath your hips. Keep your shoulder relaxed, back and down, with your arms by your side.

2. Bring one leg behind you, holding onto your foot, pulling it as close to your buttocks as comfortable.

3. Try to keep your knees next to each other while ensuring that you maintain your straight posture throughout the exercise.

4. Hold this position for 30 to 60 seconds and then change legs.

Hip Flexion Stretch

1. Begin by sitting upright on a chair with your shoulders relaxed, back and down. Keep your feet flat on the floor. Your hands can be on your lap.

2. Lift one leg up to your chest, bending at the knee, and hug your leg.

3. Hold this position for 30 to 60 seconds and then change legs.

4. Ensure your shoulders are back and down throughout the exercise.

Hip Lateral Rotation Stretch

1. Begin by sitting upright towards the front of your chair with your shoulders relaxed, back and down. Keep your feet flat on the floor. Your hands can be on your lap.

2. Straighten both of your legs in front of you and cross one leg over the other leg.

3. In a slow and controlled way, slide your heel up your shin until over the kneecap.

4. Now bend your opposite leg up, keeping your back straight and placing your hands on your shins.

5. Stay in this position, and to add a little more stretch, you can lean forward, keeping your chest up and your shoulders parallel to the floor.

6. Hold this position for 30 to 60 seconds and then change legs.

Lumbar Flexion Stretch

1. Begin by sitting upright towards the front of your chair with your shoulders relaxed, back and down. Keep your feet flat on the floor and slightly out in front of you. Your hands can be on your lap.

2. Slowly and carefully slide your hands down your legs to your feet.

3. Hold this position for 30 to 60 seconds and return to your starting position.

Lumbar Side Stretch

1. Begin by sitting upright towards the front of your chair with your shoulders relaxed, back and down. Keep your feet flat on the floor and slightly out in front of you. Your hands can be on your lap.

2. Put one of your hands behind your head, and your other hand can be left hanging straight beside you.

3. Slowly lean down to the side with the straight arm until you can feel a stretch on the opposite side. (If it is uncomfortable to place your hand on your hand behind your head, you can keep it on your lap).

Yoga Cool-Down

Cobblers Pose

1. Begin by sitting on the floor with your legs stretched out in front of you.

2. Slowly bend your knees and bring the soles of your feet together. Let your knees drop out to your sides. Your feet should be pulled in close to your groin.

3. Take hold of your feet with your hands while keeping your back straight.

4. Sit up tall, activate your midline, and make sure your shoulders are relaxed and away from your ears.

5. Breathe and relax by taking several deep breaths, gently pressing your thighs towards the floor to deepen the stretch.

6. Hold this position for 30 seconds to 1 minute, breathing deeply throughout.

7. To release this pose, slowly let go of your feet and extend your legs back out in front of you.

Sphinx Pose

Here are step-by-step instructions on how to perform the Sphinx Pose:

1. Begin by lying on your stomach with your legs extended behind you, feet hip-width apart.

2. Place your elbows directly under your shoulders and keep your forearms on the ground; your fingers should be pointing forward.

3. Keep your body aligned by keeping your legs and feet together and pressing the tops of your feet into the floor.

4. Gently lift your chest off the ground while keeping your pelvis and lower body on the floor.

5. Lengthen your spine and activate your back muscles, drawing your shoulder blades down and together, and lengthen your neck.

6. Keep your gaze forward and keep looking slightly ahead; your chin should be parallel to the floor.

7. Take deep breaths, holding the pose for 30 seconds to 1 minute, feeling the stretch in your lower back.

8. When you are ready to release the pose, you can slowly lower your chest back down to the ground.

High Alter Side Lean

1. Begin by standing tall with your feet hip-width apart and arms resting at your sides. Relax your shoulders and keep them back and down.

2. Breathe in and lift your arms over your head, bringing your palms together.

3. Firmly plant your feet into the ground, ensuring your weight is evenly distributed.

4. Breathe out and gently lean your torso to the right, keeping your hips and legs stable. Your left side should stretch.

5. Keep your arms overhead and keep a straight line from your fingertips to your toes on the left side.

6. Take deep breaths and hold the position for about 15 to 30 seconds, feeling the stretch along your left side.

7. When you are ready to release, breathe in return to an upright position, bringing your arms back to the center.

8. Breathe out and lean to the left side, repeating the stretch for another 15-30 seconds.

9. Return to the starting position, lowering your arms to your sides.

Torso Circles

1. Begin by standing with your feet shoulder-width apart and your knees slightly bent. Place your hands on your hips.

2. Activate your core muscles to maintain stability throughout the movement.

3. Breathe in, and as you exhale, gently lean your torso forward.

4. Start making a circular motion with your torso by moving to the right side, allowing your hips to follow.

5. Move your torso back, then lean to the left side, completing the circle.

6. Continue making circles in the same direction for about 5 to 10 repetitions, keeping your movements smooth and controlled.

7. After completing the circles in one direction, switch and perform the circles in the opposite direction for another 5-10 repetitions.

Cat/Cow

1. Begin by getting on your hands and knees on the floor. Use a yoga mat to keep you comfortable. Place your hands directly under your shoulders and your knees under your hips.

2. As you breathe in, arch your back, lift your tailbone, and drop your belly towards the floor. Gaze slightly upward, opening your chest. This is a cat.

3. As you breathe out, round your back towards the ceiling, tucking your chin to your chest and pulling your belly button towards your spine. This is a cow.

4. Continue to alternate between Cow Pose and Cat Pose, inhaling as you move into Cow and exhaling as you move into Cat.

5. Perform this for 5 to 10 cycles, synchronizing your breath with your movements.

6. After your last Cat Pose, return to a neutral tabletop position and take a few deep breaths.

Warrior Pose I

1. Stand with your feet together and your arms at your sides.

2. Breathe in and step your left foot back about 3 to 4 feet while keeping your right foot forward. Your right knee should be directly above your right ankle.

3. Turn your left foot at a 45-degree angle, making sure that your left heel is grounded.

4. Breathe in and lift your arms overhead, keeping them parallel to each other and your palms facing each other.

5. Activate your midline as you tuck your pelvis in slightly.

6. Turn your gaze forward by looking straight ahead and focusing on a point in front of you.

7. Keep your right knee bent and your back leg strong, holding the pose for 20 to 30 seconds while breathing deeply.

8. When you are ready to exit, breathe out and lower your arms back to your sides. Step your left foot forward to meet your right foot.

9. Perform the pose on the other side by stepping your right foot back and repeating the steps.

Warrior II

1. Begin in a standing position with your feet together and arms at your sides.

2. Breathe in and step your left foot back about 3 to 4 feet while keeping your right foot forward. Your right knee should be directly above your right ankle.

3. Turn your left foot at a 45-degree angle, making sure that your left heel is grounded.

4. Pivot your hips to face the side of your mat, aligning your torso over your pelvis.

5. Breathe out and lift your arms to the sides, parallel to the floor. Your palms should be face down.

6. Look over your right fingertips, maintaining a steady focus.

7. Keep your right knee bent and your left leg straight, holding the pose for 20 to 30 seconds while breathing deeply.

8. To release the pose, breathe in and lower your arms back to your sides. Step your left foot forward to meet your right foot.

9. Perform the pose on the opposite side by stepping your right foot back and repeating the steps.

Childs Pose

1. Begin in a kneeling position on your yoga mat with your big toes touching and knees spread apart about hip-width distance.

2. Breathe out and sit back on your heels, allowing your hips to rest toward your heels.

3. Breathe out and extend your arms forward, resting your forehead on the mat. Alternatively, you can also place your arms alongside your body with palms facing up.

4. Allow your shoulders to soften and relax into the pose.

5. Take slow, deep breaths, feeling the stretch in your back and hips as you relax deeper into the pose.

6. You can stay in this pose for 30 seconds to a few minutes. The duration will depend on your comfort level.

7. To come out of the pose, gently lift your head off the mat and walk your hands back towards your body, coming back to a seated position.

Breathe Easy: Relaxation Techniques

Pursed Lip Breathing

Here's a step-by-step breakdown of how to perform pursed-lip breathing:

1. Find a comfortable place to sit or stand. Relax your shoulders and take a moment to settle in.

2. Breathe in slowly through your nose for about two counts. Focus on filling your lungs with air.

3. Purse your lips as you prepare to exhale. Pretend that you are going to whistle. Make sure your lips are tight but not overly tense.

4. Breathe out gently through your pursed lips for about four counts. Try to make your exhalation longer than your inhalation.

5. Continue this breathing practice for several minutes. Inhale for two counts, then exhale for four counts, maintaining a steady rhythm.

6. Concentrate on breathing and counting to help keep your mind calm and focused.

7. When you're ready, return to your normal breathing pattern, taking note of how your body feels.

Diaphragmatic Breathing

Here's a step-by-step breakdown of how to perform diaphragmatic breathing:

1. Find a comfortable position, either sitting or lying down. If you're lying down, you can place a pillow under your head and your knees.

2. Put one hand on your chest and the other on your stomach. This will help you feel the movement of your diaphragm as you breathe.

3. Breathe in deeply through your nose. Focus on allowing your diaphragm to expand, pushing your stomach out while keeping your chest as still as possible.

4. After breathing in, hold your breath for about 2 to 3 seconds. This can help increase your oxygen intake.

5. Slowly breathe out through your mouth (or nose, if you prefer), allowing your stomach to fall. Imagine letting all the air out and feeling your diaphragm contract.

6. Continue this breathing practice for several minutes, focusing on deep, rhythmic breaths. Breathe in deeply, hold, and then exhale slowly.

7. Pay attention to the rise and fall of your stomach, ensuring that your chest remains relatively still. This will help activate your diaphragm.

8. When you are ready, transition back to your normal breathing pattern.

Lion's Breathe

1. Begin by sitting in a comfortable position, either on your knees or cross-legged. Keep your back straight and shoulders relaxed.

2. Take a moment to close your eyes and take a few deep breaths to relax your body and mind.

3. Breathe deeply through your nose, filling your lungs with air. As you prepare to breathe out, open your mouth wide.

4. As you breathe out, stick your tongue out toward your chin, making a "roaring" sound like a lion. Let your breath flow out forcefully.

5. Relax your face and return to a neutral position. Breathe again through your nose, preparing for the next breath.

6. Perform the Lion's Breath several times, typically around 3 to 5 times. Focus on the sound and the feeling of releasing tension.

7. After completing the breaths, close your eyes again and take a few deep, calming breaths to re-center yourself.

Alternate Nostril Breathing

1. Begin by sitting in a comfortable position with your back straight. You can also sit cross-legged on the floor or in a chair with your feet flat.

2. Bring your right hand up to your face. You can use your thumb and ring finger for this technique.

3. Use your right thumb to gently close your right nostril.

4. Inhale deeply and slowly through your left nostril for a count of four or until your lungs are comfortably full.

5. After inhaling, close your left nostril with your ring finger while releasing your right nostril.

6. Breathe out slowly and completely through your right nostril.

7. Breathe deeply through your right nostril.

8. Close your right nostril with your thumb while releasing your left nostril.

9. Breathe out slowly through your left nostril.

10. Continue this breathing practice for several minutes, alternating nostrils after each breathe-in. Aim for about 5 to 10 cycles.

11. After completing the cycles, take a few deep breaths through both nostrils and return to your normal breathing.

Equal Breathing

1. Sit or lie down in a comfortable position with your back straight. You can close your eyes if you'd like.

2. Take a deep breath through your nose for a count of four. Focus on filling your lungs and expanding your abdomen.

3. At the end of your breath in, pause for a moment.

4. Breathe out slowly through your nose for a count of four. Ensure that the exhalation is steady and controlled.

5. After breathing out, pause for a brief moment before breathing in again.

6. Continue this pattern of inhaling for four counts, holding briefly, exhaling for four counts, and pausing. Aim to maintain an equal breath throughout each cycle.

7. Concentrate on your breath and the rhythm you've established. Allow your mind to calm as you continue this practice.

8. After several minutes, slowly return to your normal breathing pattern and take a moment to notice how you feel.

Sitali Breathing

1. Sit in a comfortable position with your back straight. You can sit cross-legged or in a chair with your feet flat on the ground.

2. Stick your tongue out and curl the sides up to form a tube (or a straw-like shape). If you can't curl your tongue, you can also keep your lips pursed.

3. Slowly breathe in through your curled tongue or pursed lips. Focus on drawing in cool air.

4. After breathing in fully, close your mouth.

5. Breathe out slowly through your nose. Allow the air to flow out naturally and gently.

6. Continue this process for several rounds, usually around 5 to 10 cycles. Inhale through the mouth, then exhale through the nose.

7. Concentrate on the cooling sensation of the air as it enters your body and the calmness that follows during the exhale.

8. After completing the rounds, take a few deep breaths in and out through your nose to transition back to your regular breathing.

Humming Bee Breath

1. Sit in a comfortable position with your back straight. You can sit cross-legged on the floor or in a chair.

2. Close your eyes and take a few deep breaths to relax your body.

3. Take a deep breath through your nose, filling your lungs completely.

4. As you exhale, keep your mouth closed and make a humming sound (like "mmm"). The sound should resonate in your head, creating a gentle vibration.

5. Pay attention to the vibrations you feel in your head and body as you hum. Allow this sensation to promote relaxation.

6. Continue the process of inhaling deeply through your nose and humming for the duration of the exhalation. Aim for about 5 to 10 cycles.

7. After completing the cycles, take a moment to sit in silence and observe how you feel.

8. When you're ready, return to your normal breathing and gently open your eyes.

Key Takeaways

- Cooling down reduces Delayed Onset Muscle Soreness (DOMS) after workouts.

- It promotes stress relief through endorphin production and relaxation techniques.

- Gradually lowering the heart rate during a cool-down helps prevent dizziness and injury.

- Consistent stretching improves flexibility and muscle recovery over time.

Chapter 6:

Beginner's Luck

Now it's time for the fun part! We are going to put together some simple routines to build confidence and strength.

The following chapter will provide you with three 15-minute workout routines: lower body, upper body, and full body. I will also include warm-ups and cool-downs for each workout.

You will notice in the following chapters that as you progress, the workouts will get longer, the exercises more challenging, and the reps higher with the inclusion of weights as well.

Start where you are at in your fitness journey and work your way up.

15-Minute Lower Body Workout

Warm-up

1. Start by sitting comfortably in a chair; your feet should be flat on the ground and underneath your hips. Keep your shoulder relaxed, back and down.

2. Hold onto the sides of the seat of your chair for balance and stability.

3. Lift your left leg with your knee bent as far as is comfortable. Place your foot down with control.

4. Repeat with the opposite leg.

5. Repeat for 90 seconds, alternating each leg as you do so.

6. Return to neutral.

7. Keep your chest up and your back straight; raise up to a standing position.

8. Lower yourself back down to your seated position.

9. Repeat for 10 repetitions.

10. Now, stand up tall. Your feet should be underneath your hips. Keep your shoulder relaxed, back and down, with your arms by your side.

11. Place your hands on your hips.

12. Gently rotate your hips in a clockwise direction. Start with small circles, and as you progress through your repetitions, expand them.

13. Rotate for 12 to 15 repetitions.

14. Return to the center and repeat in an anticlockwise direction.

15. Now lift your left foot off the floor, using the chair or counter for support.

16. Gently swing your leg outwards in circles. Start with small circles, and as you progress through your repetitions, expand them.

17. Rotate for 20 repetitions.

18. Rotate in the other direction for 20 repetitions.

19. Swap legs and repeat.

The Workout

Perform 2 sets of 8 repetitions each of **Partial/Half Squat**.

1. Start by standing up tall next to a chair or counter if you need support. Keep your shoulders relaxed, back and down.

2. Your feet should be shoulder-width apart, with your toes either facing forward or slightly outwards.

3. You can hold onto the chair for support or raise your arms in front of you.

4. Activate your midline carefully, bend your hips, and sit back as you would if you were to sit on a chair.

5. As you sit back, keep your chest up and your core tight, and go no lower than 45 degrees.

6. As you stand back up, put equal weight through both legs, ensuring your feet stay flat on the floor throughout.

7. Make sure your knees stay in the line of your toes and that they don't go forward past them. Ensure that they aren't moving inward throughout the exercise.

8. Repeat for 8 repetitions.

*Rest 2 minutes between your sets.

Perform 3 sets of 5 repetitions per leg for each of **Chair Knee Extensions**.

1. Start by sitting comfortably in a chair; your feet should be flat on the ground and underneath your hips. Keep your shoulder relaxed, back and down.

2. Life up one of your legs, extending at the knee.

3. Pause and hold this position for a breath at the top of the movement, squeezing the muscles at the front of the thigh before lowering your leg back down.

4. Keep your movements controlled and slow.

5. Lower your leg, swap sides, and repeat.

6. Alternate legs and repeat for the 5 repetitions per leg.

*Rest 2 minutes between your sets.

Perform 3 sets of 5 repetitions per leg each of **Chair Knee Flexion**.

1. Start by sitting comfortably in a chair; your feet should be flat on the ground and underneath your hips. Keep your shoulder relaxed, back and down. Move towards the front of your seat.

2. Bring your left foot back towards your chair as far as it can go.

3. Return to the start position and repeat with your right foot.

4. Alternate legs and repeat for 5 repetitions.

*Rest 2 minutes between your sets.

Cool-Down

1. Start by standing up tall next to a chair or counter for support. Your feet should be underneath your hips. Keep your shoulder relaxed, back and down, with your arms by your side.

2. Place one foot out in front of you while keeping your knees straight and keeping your heels on the floor at all times.

3. Slightly bend your back knee and keep your toes facing forward.

4. Keeping your hips square and your back straight, lean forward, feeling the stretch in the back of your leg.

5. Hold this position for 30 to 60 seconds and then change legs.

6. Place one foot behind you, making sure your toes are facing forward throughout the exercise.

7. Now, bring your front knee towards the chair, ensuring that your heels remain in contact with the floor at all times.

8. Hold this position for 30 to 60 seconds and then change legs.

9. Bring one leg behind you, holding onto your foot, pulling it as close to your buttocks as comfortable.

10. Try to keep your knees next to each other while ensuring that you maintain your straight posture throughout the exercise.

11. Hold this position for 30 to 60 seconds and then change legs.

12. Move into a kneeling position on your yoga mat with your big toes touching and knees spread apart about hip-width distance.

13. Breathe out and sit back on your heels, allowing your hips to rest toward your heels.

14. Breathe out and extend your arms forward, resting your forehead on the mat. Alternatively, you can also place your arms alongside your body with palms facing up.

15. Allow your shoulders to soften and relax into the pose.

16. Take slow, deep breaths, feeling the stretch in your back and hips as you relax deeper into the pose.

17. Stay in this pose for 30 seconds to a few minutes, depending on your comfort level.

18. To come out of the pose, gently lift your head off the mat and walk your hands back towards your body, coming back to a seated position.

15-Minute Upper Body Workout

Warm-up

1. Start by standing tall. Your feet should be about shoulder-width apart. Keep your shoulder relaxed, back and down, with your arms by your side.

2. Step forward with your right leg and raise your left knee towards your chest. You can use a wall or counter for balance if you need to.

3. Using both hands or your free hand, pull your knee up close to your chest.

4. Hold for a breath and then lower the leg.

5. Repeat on the other side.

6. Alternate for the 90 seconds.

7. Gently shrug your shoulders up towards your ears.

8. Roll them back down as you squeeze your shoulder blades together.

9. Roll them towards the front and back up towards your ears.

10. Repeat for 10 rotations.

11. Roll them in the opposite direction.

12. Let your arms hang down to the side with your palms turned towards your body and thumbs facing the front.

13. Gently lift your arms up as high as you feel comfortable, pause, and then lower them back down to the sides of your body.

14. The key is to keep an upright posture throughout this exercise.

15. Repeat for 10 repetitions.

16. Slowly look over your shoulder to the side.

17. Pause for a breath and return to the center.

18. Slowly look over your other shoulder.

19. Pause for a breath and return to the center.

20. Repeat for 10 repetitions.

The Workout

Perform 3 sets of 5 of **Wall Push-Ups.**

1. Begin by facing a wall with your feet a little more than shoulder-width apart.

2. Position your hands by extending your arms in front of you and placing your palms flat against the wall at shoulder height. Your hands should be slightly wider than your shoulders.

3. Take a few steps back from the wall so that your body is at an angle. Your feet should be placed firmly on the ground.

4. Activate your core by tightening your abdominal muscles to support your lower back.

5. Breathe in as you bend your elbows to slowly lower your chest towards the wall. Keep your body straight and aligned from the top of your head to your feet.

6. Exhale as you straighten your arms to push your body back to the starting position.

7. Repeat for 5 repetitions.

*Rest 90 seconds between each set.

Perform 3 sets of 8 reps of **Seated Row**.

1. Start by sitting comfortably in a chair; your feet should be flat on the ground and underneath your hips. Keep your shoulder relaxed, back and down.
2. Make a fist with both of your hands and extend your arms out in front of you.
3. Pull your elbows back behind you as you squeeze your shoulder blades together at the end of the movement.
4. Remember to keep your chest up throughout this exercise.
5. Repeat for 8 repetitions.

*Rest 90 seconds between each set.

Perform 3 sets of 5 reps of **Tricep Lifts**.

1. Start by sitting comfortably towards the front of your chair, and your feet should be flat on the ground and underneath your hips. Keep your shoulder relaxed, back and down.
2. Put your hands on either side of the seat of the chair near your hips or on the armrests.
3. Bend slightly forward at the hips while keeping your back straight.
4. Now press through your hands, straightening your elbows and lifting your buttocks off the chair, if you can.
5. Slowly lower your buttocks back to the chair by bending at your elbows.
6. Repeat for 5 repetitions.

*Rest 90 seconds between each set.

Cool-Down

1. Start by standing up tall or, if you prefer, sitting down comfortably in a chair.

2. Your feet should be placed underneath your hips.

3. Cross your arms over your chest and gently rotate around until you feel a stretch in your upper back.

4. Hold this position for 30 to 60 seconds and repeat on the opposite side.

5. Interlace your fingers and turn your palms away from you.

6. Raise your arms up above your head, towards the ceiling, and push-up as far as you can.

7. Hold this position for 30 to 60 seconds.

8. Raise your arms straight up in front of you, parallel to the floor.

9. Now, bring your arms out to the side, pulling as far back as you can and squeezing your shoulder blades together while keeping your posture upright.

10. If you have difficulty holding your arms at 90 degrees (or parallel to the floor), you can hold your arms lower (45 degrees).

11. Hold this position for 30 to 60 seconds.

12. Breathe in and lift your arms over your head, bringing your palms together.

13. Firmly plant your feet into the ground, ensuring your weight is evenly distributed.

14. Breathe out and gently lean your torso to the right, keeping your hips and legs stable. Your left side should stretch.

15. Keep your arms overhead and keep a straight line from your fingertips to your toes on the left side.

16. Take deep breaths and hold the position for about 15 to 30 seconds, feeling the stretch along your left side.

17. When you are ready to release, breathe in return to an upright position, bringing your arms back to the center.

18. Breathe out and lean to the left side, repeating the stretch for another 15 to 30 seconds.

19. Return to the starting position, lowering your arms to your sides.

15-Minute Full-Body Workout

Warm-up

1. Start by standing up tall, and your feet should be underneath your hips. Keep your shoulder relaxed, back and down, with your arms by your side.

2. Begin marching by lifting your right knee up towards your waist. Try to keep your knee in line with your hip.

3. As you lift your knee, swing your left arm forward and your right arm back. This will create a marching rhythm.

4. Lower your right leg and lift your left knee while swinging your right arm forward and your left arm back.

5. Continue alternating legs and arms for 30 to 60 seconds.

6. Raise your arms out to the side of you at shoulder height. Your palms should be facing downward.

7. Rotate your arms forward in circles. Start with small circles, and as you progress through your repetitions, expand them.

8. Rotate for 20 repetitions.

9. Rotate in the other direction for 20 repetitions.

10. Lift your left foot off the floor, using the chair or counter for support.

11. Gently swing your leg outwards in circles. Start with small circles, and as you progress through your repetitions, expand them.

12. Rotate for 20 repetitions.

13. Rotate in the other direction for 20 repetitions.

14. Swap legs and repeat.

15. Get down on your hands and knees on the floor, and use a yoga mat to keep you comfortable. Place your hands directly under your shoulders and your knees under your hips.

16. Activate your abdominal muscles to stabilize your torso and keep your back flat and your spine in a neutral position.

17. Slowly reach your right arm forward, extending it straight in front of you at shoulder height. At the same time, extend your left leg straight back, keeping it in line with your body and parallel to the floor.

18. Pause for a breath, focusing on your balance.

19. Return to your starting position by lowering your right arm and left leg back to the floor so that you are on all fours again.

20. Repeat the movement by extending your left arm forward and right leg back, following the same process.

21. Continue to alternate between sides for the stipulated amount of repetitions.

The Workout

Perform 2 sets of 3 of **Inchworms**.

1. Start by standing tall. Your feet should be about shoulder-width apart. Keep your shoulders relaxed, back and down, with your arms by your side.

2. Bend at your waist and reach down towards the ground, trying to keep your legs straight. If you can't touch the ground, it's okay to bend your knees slightly.

3. Place your hands on the ground in front of you and walk them forward until you are in a plank position (hands under your shoulders, body in a straight line).

4. Keep your core engaged to ensure your body stays straight and stable.

5. Take small steps to walk your feet towards your hands, keeping your legs as straight as possible. This will bring you back into a standing position.

6. Once you are back in the starting position, bend forward again and repeat the movement.

7. Repeat for 3 repetitions.

*Rest 90 seconds between each set.

Perform 3 sets of 5 of **Squat to Overhead Press**.

1. Start by standing up tall. Keep your shoulders relaxed, back and down. Clench your fists, hold them at the front of your shoulders with your palms facing each other, and elbows bent.

2. Your feet should be shoulder-width apart, with your toes either facing forward or slightly outwards.

3. Lower your body into a squat by bending at your hips and sitting back as you would if you were to sit on a chair. Make sure your knees stay in the line of your toes; they don't go forward past your toes, and they aren't moving inward throughout the exercise.

4. As you sit back, keep your chest up and your core tight; aim to go to 90 degrees or slightly lower.

5. As you reach the bottom of the squat (thighs parallel to the ground or lower), transition to the overhead press position by keeping your fists at your shoulders.

6. As you stand back up, put equal weight through both legs, ensuring your feet stay flat on the floor throughout while lifting your fists overhead by extending your arms fully overhead as you stand upright, ensuring your elbows are locked at the top.

7. Lower your hands back to shoulder height as you prepare for the next squat.

8. Repeat for 5 repetitions.

*Rest 90 seconds between each set.

Perform 3 sets of 30 seconds of **Farmers Carry**.

1. Start by standing up tall. Keep your shoulders relaxed, back and down. Stand with your feet shoulder-width apart, holding a dumbbell or kettlebell in both hands at your side.

2. Activate your midline to maintain stability and posture throughout the movement.

3. Keep your shoulders back and chest up, ensuring your body is straight.

4. Begin walking forward, taking small, controlled steps while maintaining your posture and balance.

5. Keep the kettlebell or dumbbell close to your body. Maintain a neutral spine and avoid hunching your shoulders.

6. Continue walking for a set distance or duration, such as 20 to 30 feet, or for a specific time, like 30 seconds to 1 minute.

7. Once you have completed your distance or time frame, switch the weight to the other hand and repeat the carry in the opposite direction.

8. Once completed, lower the weight safely to the ground.

*Rest 60 seconds between each set.

Cool-Down

1. Start by standing up tall or, if you prefer, sitting down comfortably in a chair.

2. Your feet should be placed underneath your hips.

3. Place one arm straight in front of your body and use your other hand to hug the straight arm to your body.

4. Hold this position for 30 to 60 seconds.

5. Release and repeat on the other side.

6. Take one large step out to the side and face your toes outwards.

7. Shift your weight to one side, bending that knee. You will feel a stretch on the inner thigh of the straight leg.

8. Hold this position for 30 to 60 seconds and then change legs.

9. Move down to the floor with your legs stretched out in front of you.

10. Carefully bend your knees and bring the soles of your feet together. Let your knees drop out to your sides. Your feet should be pulled in close to your groin.

11. Take hold of your feet with your hands while keeping your back straight.

12. Sit up tall, activate your midline, and make sure your shoulders are relaxed and away from your ears.

13. Breathe and relax by taking several deep breaths, gently pressing your thighs towards the floor to deepen the stretch.

14. Hold this position for 30 seconds to 1 minute, breathing deeply throughout.

15. To release this pose, slowly let go of your feet and extend your legs back out in front of you.

16. Now lie down on your stomach with your legs extended behind you, feet hip-width apart.

17. Place your elbows directly under your shoulders and keep your forearms on the ground; your fingers should be pointing forward.

18. Keep your body aligned by keeping your legs and feet together and pressing the tops of your feet into the floor.

19. Gently lift your chest off the ground while keeping your pelvis and lower body on the floor.

20. Lengthen your spine and activate your back muscles, drawing your shoulder blades down and together, and lengthen your neck.

21. Keep your gaze forward and keep looking slightly ahead; your chin should be parallel to the floor.

22. Take deep breaths, holding the pose for 30 seconds to 1 minute, feeling the stretch in your lower back.

23. When you are ready to release the pose, you can slowly lower your chest back down to the ground.

Chapter 7:

Midway Marvels

Congrats, you are ready to step up your game. The next workout routine will be 30 minutes long with slightly more challenging bodyweight exercises.

I will provide you with an upper body, lower body, and full-body workout. As with the previous chapter, there will also be a warm-up and cool-down.

30-Minute Lower Body Workout

Warm-up

1. Start by standing up tall, and your feet should be underneath your hips. Keep your shoulder relaxed, back and down, with your arms by your side.

2. Raise your arms out to the sides and overhead and jump or step your feet out so they're slightly more than shoulder-width apart.

3. Without pausing, quickly bring your arms back down to your side and your feet together.

4. Repeat for 30 to 60 seconds.

5. Rest for 1 minute and repeat.

6. Stand up tall next to your chair or counter for support. Your feet should be underneath your hips. Keep your shoulder relaxed, back and down, with your arms by your side.

7. Lift your left foot off the floor, using the chair or counter for support.

8. Gently swing your leg outwards in circles. Start with small circles, and as you progress through your repetitions, expand them.

9. Rotate for 20 repetitions.

10. Rotate in the other direction for 20 repetitions.

11. Swap legs and repeat.

12. Start by standing tall. Your feet should be about shoulder-width apart. Keep your shoulder relaxed, back and down, with your arms by your side.

13. Gently bend down until your hands touch the flow.

14. Carefully and slowly walk your hands forward until you get into a plank position or as far as comfortable.

15. Pause for a second, then walk your hands back toward your feet.

16. Return to standing.

17. Continue for 30 to 60 seconds.

18. Rest for 2 minutes and repeat.

The Workout

Perform 3 sets of 8 repetitions each of **Squat**.

1. Start by standing up tall next to a chair or counter if you need support. Keep your shoulders relaxed, back and down.

2. Your feet should be shoulder-width apart, with your toes either facing forward or slightly outwards.

3. You can hold onto the chair for support or raise your arms in front of you.

4. Activate your midline carefully, bend your hips, and sit back as you would if you were to sit on a chair.

5. As you sit back, keep your chest up and your core tight; aim to go to 90 degrees or slightly lower.

6. As you stand back up, put equal weight through both legs, ensuring your feet stay flat on the floor throughout.

7. Make sure your knees stay in the line of your toes; they don't go forward past your toes, and they aren't moving inward throughout the exercise.

8. Repeat for 8 repetitions.

*Rest 1 minute between sets.

Perform 3 sets of 15 repetitions each of **Glute Bridges**.

1. Begin by lying on your back on a mat or flat surface with your knees bent and feet flat on the floor, hip-width apart. Your arms should be at your sides, palms facing down.

2. Keep your feet close to your glutes so that they are within comfortable reaching distance.

3. Before lifting your hips, activate your midline and stabilize your core muscles.

4. Press through your heels and squeeze your glutes as you carefully lift your hips off the ground.

5. Keep your back straight, and try not to overarch and hyperextend excessively.

6. Raise your hips until your body forms a straight line from your shoulders to your knees, and hold this position for a breath while you focus on squeezing your glutes.

7. When you are finished, carefully lower your hips back down to the floor. Make sure that you control the movement as you do so.

8. Repeat for the 15 repetitions.

*Rest 90 seconds minute between sets.

Perform 3 sets of 12 repetitions each of **Side Leg Raises**.

1. Begin by lying on your side on a mat or flat surface with your knees bent and feet flat on the floor, hip-width apart. You can either rest your head on your arm or place a cushion under your head to make yourself comfortable.

2. Keep your body in a straight line from your head to your feet, with your legs stacked on top of each other.

3. Bend your bottom leg at your knee while keeping it flat on the ground to keep you stable. You can also keep it straight if you prefer.

4. Keep your top leg straight as you slowly lift it up toward the ceiling. Activate your glutes and midline as you raise your leg.

5. Lift your leg till it is about 45 degrees off the ground or as high as you feel comfortable. Hold this position for a breath while making sure your body remains in a straight line.

6. Slowly lower your leg back down to the starting position.

7. Repeat for 12 repetitions on one side, then swap sides and repeat on the other.

*Rest 90 seconds minute between sets.

Perform 3 sets of 30 seconds of **Cobra**.

1. Begin by lying face down on the floor. Use a yoga mat to keep you comfortable. Place your hands directly under your shoulders and hands facing forward. Extend your legs and point your toes away from your body.

2. Breathe out, press your hips into the mat or floor, and push your chest upwards and away from the floor while keeping your hips on the ground. Your arms should extend fully.

3. This will arch your lower back and you will feel a stretch in the muscles in your chest and abs. Hold this position for 15 to 30 seconds.

4. When you are ready to release, slowly lower your chest back to the floor.

*Rest 1 minute between sets.

Perform 3 sets of 15 seconds of **Plank**.

1. Begin by getting on your hands and knees on the floor. Use a yoga mat to keep you comfortable. Place your hands directly under your shoulders and your knees under your hips.

2. Your hands should be placed slightly wider than shoulder-width apart and your feet together. Tuck your toes under and lift your body off the ground, creating a straight line from your head to your heels.

3. Engage your abdominal muscles, core muscles, glutes, and legs to maintain a stable position and prevent your hips from dropping.

4. Keep your head in a neutral position, looking at the floor slightly ahead of your hands. Avoid tilting your head up or dropping it down.

5. Maintain this position for 15 seconds, focusing on your breathing and staying relaxed.

6. When you are ready to release the hold, gently lower your knees to the ground and return to a resting position.

*Rest 1 minute between sets.

Cool-Down

1. Start by standing up tall next to a chair or counter for support. Your feet should be underneath your hips. Keep your shoulder relaxed, back and down, with your arms by your side.

2. Bring one leg behind you, holding onto your foot, pulling it as close to your buttocks as comfortable.

3. Try to keep your knees next to each other while ensuring that you maintain your straight posture throughout the exercise.

4. Hold this position for 30 to 60 seconds and then change legs.

5. Now sit up straight on a chair with your shoulders relaxed, back and down. Keep your feet flat on the floor. Your hands can be on your lap.

6. Lift one leg up to your chest, bending at the knee, and hug your leg.

7. Hold this position for 30 to 60 seconds and then change legs.

8. Ensure your shoulders are back and down throughout the exercise.

9. Now, straighten both of your legs in front of you and cross one leg over the other leg.

10. In a slow and controlled way, slide your heel up your shin until over the kneecap.

11. Now bend your opposite leg up while keeping your back straight. Place your hands on your shins.

12. Stay in this position, and to add a little more stretch, you can lean forward, keeping your chest up and your shoulders parallel to the floor.

13. Hold this position for 30 to 60 seconds and then change legs.

14. Slowly and carefully slide your hands down your legs to your feet.

15. Hold this position for 30 to 60 seconds and return to your starting position.

16. Now stand up and stand with your feet together and your arms at your sides.

17. Breathe in and step your left foot back about 3 to 4 feet while keeping your right foot forward. Your right knee should be directly above your right ankle.

18. Turn your left foot at a 45-degree angle, making sure that your left heel is grounded.

19. Breathe in and lift your arms overhead, keeping them parallel to each other and your palms facing each other.

20. Activate your midline as you tuck your pelvis in slightly.

21. Turn your gaze forward by looking straight ahead and focusing on a point in front of you.

22. Keep your right knee bent and your back leg strong, holding the pose for 20 to 30 seconds while breathing deeply.

23. When you are ready to exit, breathe out and lower your arms back to your sides. Step your left foot forward to meet your right foot.

24. Perform the pose on the other side by stepping your right foot back and repeating the steps.

30-Minute Upper Body Workout

Warm-up

1. Start by standing up tall; your feet should be underneath your hips. Keep your shoulder relaxed, back and down, with your arms by your side.

2. Gently squat down by bending your knees and lowering your body into a squat position; place your hands on the floor in front of you.

3. Walk your feet back while keeping your hands on the ground. Your body should be in a straight line from your head to your heels (this is the plank position).

4. If you are able to, carefully lower your body towards the ground by bending your elbows and doing one push-up.

5. Walk or jump your feet back toward your hands to return to the squat position.

6. Stand or jump up as you reach your hands overhead.

7. Return to the starting position.

8. Repeat for 5 repetitions.

9. Rest for 1 minute and repeat for another 5 repetitions.

10. Now, stand up tall.

11. Your feet should be placed underneath your hips.

12. Gently shrug your shoulders up towards your ears.

13. Roll them back down as you squeeze your shoulder blades together.

14. Roll them towards the front and back up towards your ears.

15. Repeat for 10 rotations.

16. Roll them in the opposite direction.

17. Place your hands on your hips, and as you do so, bring your shoulders forward, which will make your upper back round.

18. Bring your shoulders back and down while pulling your elbows back and squeezing your shoulder blades together.

19. The key here is to keep your shoulders down throughout this exercise.

20. Repeat for 10 repetitions.

21. Bring your left ear to your left shoulder, as far as you feel comfortable.

22. Try not to lift your shoulder to your ear.

23. Hold this stretch for 30 to 60 seconds as you focus on relaxing your neck.

24. Repeat on the other side.

25. Raise your arms out to the side of you at shoulder height. Your palms should be facing downward.

26. Keeping your arms straight, swing both arms towards each other until they cross in front of your chest.

27. Swing them out to your side again. Repeat this, alternating between which arm is on top of the other during crossover.

28. Repeat for 20 repetitions.

29. Raise your arms out to the sides, just below shoulder height.

30. Bend your elbows as if trying to put your fingertips on your shoulders.

31. Begin making small circles in the air with the tips of your bent elbows.

32. Repeat for 10 rotations.

33. Roll them in the opposite direction.

34. Now position yourself with your back against a wall with your heels about 6 inches away. You should be standing up tall; your feet should be underneath your hips.

35. Press your lower back, upper back, and head against the wall. Keep your feet flat on the floor.

36. Raise your arms to your side, bending at a 90-degree angle, with your elbows at shoulder height and your fingers pointed upward. Your upper arms should be against the wall.

37. Slowly slide your arms upward along the wall, keeping contact with the wall throughout the movement. Your arms should straightened fully by the time your hands reach above your head.

38. Lower your arms by reversing the movement. Lower your arms back down to the starting position, keeping your elbows and wrists in contact with the wall as you do so.

39. Repeat for 12 repetitions.

The Workout

Perform 3 sets of 8 repetitions each of the **Chair Push-Ups**.

1. Start by standing up tall next to a chair and placing both hands on the backrest. Your feet should be underneath your hips. Make sure your chair is stable and will not slide.

2. Bend forward from your hips while keeping your back straight and your abdominal muscles activated.

3. Keep a slight bend in your knees you bend your elbows and bring your chest towards the chair.

4. Now, straighten your arms, bringing your chest away from the chair, and repeat for the set repetitions.

*Rest for 90 seconds between sets.

Perform 3 sets of 8 repetitions of each of the **Tricep Lifts**.

1. Start by sitting comfortably towards the front of your chair; your feet should be flat on the ground and underneath your hips. Keep your shoulder relaxed, back and down.

2. Put your hands on either side of the seat of the chair near your hips or on the armrests.

3. Lean slightly forward at the hips while keeping your back straight.

4. Now press through your hands, straightening your elbows and lifting your buttocks off the chair, if you can.

5. Slowly lower your buttocks back to the chair by bending at your elbows.

6. Repeat for 8 repetitions.

*Rest for 90 seconds between sets.

Perform 3 sets of 6 repetitions on each arm of **Shoulder Taps**.

1. Begin by getting on your hands and knees on the floor. Use a yoga mat to keep you comfortable. Place your hands directly under your shoulders and your knees under your hips.

2. Start in a high plank with your palms flat, hands shoulder-width apart, shoulders stacked directly above your wrists, but keep your knees on the floor and raise your upper body only.

3. Tap your right hand to your left shoulder while keeping your core and glutes activated and trying to keep your hips as still as possible.

4. Do the same thing with your left hand to your right shoulder. That's 1 rep.

5. Repeat for 6 reps on each arm, alternating sides.

*Rest for 2 minutes between sets.

Perform 3 sets of 12 repetitions on each arm of **Crunch**.

1. Begin by lying on your back. Use a yoga mat to keep you comfortable. Bend your knees and keep your feet flat on the ground with your heels 12 to 18 away from you.

2. Place your hands behind your head for support. You will keep this position throughout the exercise.

3. Breathe out as you activate your midline and bring your chin slightly towards your chest. Curl your torso towards your thighs.

4. Keep your neck relaxed and keep your chin towards your chest. Your feet and lower back stay on the floor throughout the whole movement. Continue to curl yourself up until your upper back lifts off the floor.

5. Hold this position briefly.

6. Return to your starting position by gently curling back down.

7. Repeat for the stipulated amount of repetitions.

*Rest for 30 seconds between sets.

Perform 1 set for as long as possible of a heavy **Suitcase Carry**.

1. Start by standing up tall. Keep your shoulders relaxed, back and down. Stand with your feet shoulder-width apart, holding a dumbbell or kettlebell in one hand at your side.

2. Activate your midline to maintain stability and posture throughout the movement.

3. Keep your shoulders back and chest up, ensuring your body is straight.

4. Begin walking forward, taking small, controlled steps while maintaining your posture and balance.

5. Keep the kettlebell or dumbbell close to your body, and avoid leaning to one side. Maintain a neutral spine and avoid hunching your shoulders.

6. Continue walking for a set distance or duration, such as 20 to 30 feet, or for a specific time, like 30 seconds to 1 minute.

7. Once you have completed your distance or time frame, switch the weight to the other hand and repeat the carry in the opposite direction.

8. Once completed, lower the weight safely to the ground.

Cool-Down

1. Start by standing up tall or, if you prefer, sitting down comfortably in a chair.

2. Your feet should be placed underneath your hips.

3. Place your arms on your thighs, or let them hang to your side.

4. Carefully lean your head straight back, looking up to the ceiling and going as far back as you feel comfortable. Do not push into any pain.

5. Hold for 30 to 60 seconds.

6. Release and return to neutral.

7. Place the hand on the side you are stretching behind the shoulder to stabilize your shoulder blade. If unable to do this, just perform the exercise without placing one hand behind your shoulder.

8. Carefully turn your head to about 45 degrees to one side and bring your head down as if you are looking at your knee on that side.

9. You will feel a stretch on the opposite side you are looking behind the neck and shoulder.

10. If you would like to increase the stretch, place your hand on the back of your head and apply gentle pressure.

11. Hold for 30 to 60 seconds.

12. Carefully return your head to the starting position.

13. Cross your arms over your chest and gently rotate around until you feel a stretch in your upper back.

14. Hold this position for 30 to 60 seconds and repeat on the opposite side.

15. Interlace your fingers and turn your palms away from you.

16. Raise your arms up above your head, towards the ceiling, and push-up as far as you can.

17. Hold this position for 30 to 60 seconds.

18. Breathe in and lift your arms over your head, bringing your palms together.

19. Firmly plant your feet into the ground, ensuring your weight is evenly distributed.

20. Breathe out and gently lean your torso to the right, keeping your hips and legs stable. Your left side should stretch.

21. Keep your arms overhead and keep a straight line from your fingertips to your toes on the left side.

22. Take deep breaths and hold the position for about 15 to 30 seconds, feeling the stretch along your left side.

23. When you are ready to release, breathe in return to an upright position, bringing your arms back to center.

24. Breathe out and lean to the left side, repeating the stretch for another 15-30 seconds.

25. Return to the starting position, lowering your arms to your sides.

30-Minute Full-Body Workout

Warm-Up

1. Start by standing up tall, and your feet should be underneath your hips. Keep your shoulder relaxed, back and down, with your arms by your side.

2. Raise your arms out to the sides and overhead and jump or step your feet out so they're slightly more than shoulder-width apart.

3. Without pausing, quickly bring your arms back down to your side and your feet together.

4. Repeat for 30 to 60 seconds.

5. Rest for 1 minute before repeating.

6. Gently bend down until your hands touch the flow.

7. Carefully and slowly walk your hands forward until you get into a plank position or as far as comfortable.

8. Pause for a second, then walk your hands back toward your feet.

9. Return to standing.

10. Continue for 30 to 60 seconds.

11. Get down on your hands and knees on the floor. Use a yoga mat to keep you comfortable. Place your hands directly under your shoulders and your knees under your hips.

12. Activate your abdominal muscles to stabilize your torso and keep your back flat and your spine in a neutral position.

13. Slowly reach your right arm forward, extending it straight in front of you at shoulder height. At the same time, extend your left leg straight back, keeping it in line with your body and parallel to the floor.

14. Pause for a breath, focusing on your balance.

15. Return to your starting position by lowering your right arm and left leg back to the floor so that you are on all fours again.

16. Repeat the movement by extending your left arm forward and right leg back, following the same process.

17. Continue to alternate between sides for 8 repetitions on each side.

18. Stand up tall.

19. Raise your arms out to the sides, just below shoulder height.

20. Bend your elbows as if trying to put your fingertips on your shoulders.

21. Begin making small circles in the air with the tips of your bent elbows.

22. Repeat for 10 rotations.

23. Roll them in the opposite direction.

24. Lift your left foot off the floor, using the chair or counter for support.

25. Gently swing your leg outwards in circles. Start with small circles, and as you progress through your repetitions, expand them.

26. Rotate for 20 repetitions.

27. Rotate in the other direction for 20 repetitions.

28. Swap legs and repeat.

The Workout

Perform 3 sets of 15 seconds of **Bear Crawl**.

1. Begin by getting on your hands and knees on the floor. Use a yoga mat to keep you comfortable. Place your hands directly under your shoulders and your knees under your hips.

2. Raise your knees off the ground a few inches while keeping your back flat. This is your starting bear crawl position.

3. Move your right hand and left foot forward at the same time, followed by your left hand and right foot. Aim to keep your body low and controlled.

4. As you move, keep your midline active and stabilize your body. You do not want your hips to sway.

5. Continue to alternate moving your hands and feet, crawling forward for 15 seconds.

*Rest for 2 minutes after each set.

Perform 3 sets of 5 repetitions of **Inchworm**.

1. Start by standing tall. Your feet should be about shoulder-width apart. Keep your shoulders relaxed, back and down, with your arms by your side.

2. Bend at your waist and reach down towards the ground, trying to keep your legs straight. If you can't touch the ground, it's okay to bend your knees slightly.

3. Place your hands on the ground in front of you and walk them forward until you are in a plank position (hands under your shoulders, body in a straight line).

4. Keep your core engaged to ensure your body stays straight and stable.

5. Take small steps to walk your feet towards your hands, keeping your legs as straight as possible. This will bring you back into a standing position.

6. Once you are back in the starting position, bend forward again and repeat the movement.

7. Repeat for 5 repetitions.

*Rest for 1 minute after each set.

Perform 3 sets of 6 repetitions on each side of **Bicycle Crunches**.

1. Begin by lying on your back. Use a yoga mat to keep you comfortable. Bend your knees and keep your feet flat on the ground with your heels 12 to 18 away from you.

2. Place your hands behind your head for support. You will keep this position throughout the exercise.

3. Carefully lift both feet off the floor, moving your knees towards your torso until your thighs align vertically to the floor, creating a 90-degree angle at your hips. Keep the 90-degree bend at the knee and relax your feet, allowing them to point away from your body.

4. Bring your right knee towards your chest in a straight line and extend your left leg while keeping it off the floor. At the same time, lift your shoulders off the floor and bring your left elbow towards your right knee.

5. Your lower back should remain pressed against the floor.

6. Do these two movements simultaneously.

7. Move carefully and slowly until your elbow touches or almost touches your opposite knee. Hold for a breath and return to the starting position.

8. Repeat on the opposite side.

9. Repeat for 6 repetitions on each side.

*Rest for 1 minute after each set.

Perform 3 sets of 12 repetitions of **Calf Raises**.

1. Start by standing up tall next to a chair or counter if you need support. Keep your shoulders relaxed, back and down.

2. Your feet should be hip-width apart.

3. Keep your knees straight and hold onto the chair for support if needed.

4. Come up onto your toes and raise your heels off the floor.

5. Hold this position briefly before lowering yourself back down.

6. Repeat for 12 repetitions.

*Rest for 1 minute after each set.

Perform 3 sets of 8 repetitions on each side of **Lateral Lunges**.

1. Start by standing tall. Your feet should be about hip-width apart. Keep your shoulders relaxed, back and down, with your hands on your hips or clasped in front of your chest.

2. Carefully take a wide step to your right with your right foot. Keep your left leg straight as you begin to bend your right knee.

3. As you step to the side, push your hips back and lower your body toward your right knee. Make sure that your right knee stays aligned with your right foot and does not extend past your toes.

4. Keep your back straight by keeping your chest up throughout the movement. Try to avoid rounding your back.

5. Lower your body until your right thigh is parallel to the ground or as low as you can comfortably go. Hold this position for one breath.

6. Push through your right foot to return to the starting position, and activate your glutes and leg muscles as you stand up.

7. Once you've completed your repetitions on the right side, repeat the movement on your left side by stepping to the left and bending your left knee while keeping your right leg straight.

8. Alternate sides for 8 repetitions on each side.

*Rest for 90 seconds after each set.

Cool-Down

1. Start by standing up tall or, if you prefer, sitting down comfortably in a chair.

2. Your feet should be placed underneath your hips.

3. Place your arms on your thighs, or let them hang to your side.

4. Look over to your left shoulder as far as you feel comfortable.

5. Hold for 30 to 60 seconds.

6. Look over to your right shoulder as far as you feel comfortable.

7. Hold for 30 to 60 seconds.

8. Carefully return your head to the starting position.

9. Bring your ear down to your shoulder; do not bring your shoulder up to your ear; leave your shoulder relaxed. Go as far as you feel comfortable.

10. To increase the stretch, place your hand on the side of your head and apply gentle pressure.

11. Hold this position for 30 to 60 seconds.

12. Place one arm straight in front of your body and use your other hand to hug the straight arm to your body.

13. Hold this position for 30 to 60 seconds.

14. Release and repeat on the other side.

15. Stand up tall next to a chair or counter for support. Your feet should be underneath your hips. Keep your shoulder relaxed, back and down, with your arms by your side.

16. Place one foot behind you, making sure your toes are facing forward throughout the exercise.

17. Now, bring your front knee towards the chair, ensuring that your heels remain in contact with the floor at all times.

18. Hold this position for 30 to 60 seconds and then change legs.

19. Bring your feet together and place your arms at your sides.

20. Breathe in and step your left foot back about 3-4 feet while keeping your right foot forward. Your right knee should be directly above your right ankle.

1. Turn your left foot at a 45-degree angle, making sure that your left heel is grounded.

2. Pivot your hips to face the side of your mat, aligning your torso over your pelvis.

3. Breathe out and lift your arms to the sides, parallel to the floor. Your palms should face down.

4. Look over your right fingertips, maintaining a steady focus.

5. Keep your right knee bent and your left leg straight, holding the pose for 20 to 30 seconds while breathing deeply.

6. To release the pose, breathe in and lower your arms back to your sides. Step your left foot forward to meet your right foot.

7. Perform the pose on the opposite side by stepping your right foot back and repeating the steps.

Chapter 8:

Advanced Aces

You have worked hard to get here! In this chapter, I will provide 45-minute workouts with more advanced movements that also may require weights, such as dumbbells or kettlebells.

Along with a warm-up and cool-down, we are also going to add quick HIIT workouts to give you a bit of a cardio challenge after your strength workout.

45-Minute Upper Body Workout

Warm-up

1. Start by standing up tall, and your feet should be underneath your hips. Keep your shoulder relaxed, back and down, with your arms by your side.

2. Gently squat down by bending your knees and lowering your body into a squat position; place your hands on the floor in front of you.

3. Walk your feet back while keeping your hands on the ground. Your body should be in a straight line from your head to your heels (this is the plank position).

4. If you are able to, carefully lower your body towards the ground by bending your elbows and doing one push-up.

5. Walk or jump your feet back toward your hands to return to the squat position.

6. Stand or jump up as you reach your hands overhead.

7. Return to the starting position.

8. Repeat for 45 seconds.

9. Rest for 90 seconds and repeat.

10. Gently shrug your shoulders up towards your ears.

11. Roll them back down as you squeeze your shoulder blades together.

12. Roll them towards the front and back up towards your ears.

13. Repeat for 10 rotations.

14. Roll them in the opposite direction.

15. Place your hands on your hips, and as you do so, bring your shoulders forward, which will make your upper back round.

16. Bring your shoulders back and down while pulling your elbows back and squeezing your shoulder blades together.

17. The key here is to keep your shoulders down throughout this exercise.

18. Repeat for 12 repetitions.

19. Bring your left ear to your left shoulder, as far as you feel comfortable.

20. Try not to lift your shoulder to your ear.

21. Hold this stretch for 30 to 60 seconds as you focus on relaxing your neck.

22. Repeat on the other side.

23. Raise your arms out to the side of you at shoulder height. Your palms should be facing downward.

24. Rotate your arms forward in circles. Start with small circles, and as you progress through your repetitions, expand them.

25. Rotate for 20 repetitions.

26. Rotate in the other direction for 20 repetitions.

27. Raise your arms out to the side of you at shoulder height. Your palms should be facing downward.

28. Keeping your arms straight swing both arms towards each other until they cross in front of your chest.

29. Swing them out to your side again. Repeat this, alternating between which arm is on top of the other during crossover.

30. Repeat for 20 repetitions.

31. Position yourself with your back against a wall with your heels about 6 inches away. You should be standing up tall, and your feet should be underneath your hips.

32. Press your lower back, upper back, and head against the wall. Keep your feet flat on the floor.

33. Raise your arms to your side, bending at a 90-degree angle, with your elbows at shoulder height and your fingers pointed upward. Your upper arms should be against the wall.

34. Slowly slide your arms upward along the wall, keeping contact with the wall throughout the movement. Your arms should straightened fully by the time your hands reach above your head.

35. Lower your arms by reversing the movement. Lower your arms back down to the starting position, keeping your elbows and wrists in contact with the wall as you do so.

36. Repeat for 10 repetitions.

The Workout

Perform 3 sets of 8 repetitions of **Push-Up**.

1. Begin by getting on your hands and knees on the floor. Use a yoga mat to keep you comfortable. Place your hands directly under your shoulders and your knees under your hips.

2. Walk your feet out so that you get into a plank position. Your hands should be placed slightly wider than shoulder-width apart and your feet together. Your body should form a straight line from the top of your head to your feet.

3. Activate your abdominal muscles to help you keep your body straight and engaged as you perform the movement.

4. Breathe in as you bend your elbows and lower yourself until your chest is just above the floor. Keep your hips in line with your body.

5. Press up through your palms to push your body back up to the starting positions with your arms straight and locked out.

6. Repeat for 8 repetitions.

*Rest for 90 seconds between sets.

Perform 3 sets of 10 repetitions on each arm of the **Bicep Curl**.

1. Start by standing up tall, and your feet should be underneath your hips.

2. Let your arms hang by your sides with your dumbbell in your hands with your palms facing forward.

3. From this position, curl your arm from the elbow all the way up until your closed fist almost touches your shoulder, and then slowly lower it back down.

4. Repeat on the other side with the other arm.

5. Repeat for 10 repetitions on each arm, alternating arms as you do so.

This exercise can also be done with both arms at the same time.

*Rest for 1 minute between sets.

Perform 3 sets of 8 repetitions of **Shoulder Press Ups**.

1. Start by standing up tall, and your feet should be underneath your hips.

2. Take hold of two dumbbells and bring your hands up to either side of your shoulders with your palms facing each other.

3. Now press up and slowly lift your hands up above your head as far as you can go, and then slowly lift them back down to the start position.

4. Make sure you do not over-arch your back as you do so.

5. Repeat for 8 repetitions.

*Rest for 2 minutes between sets.

Perform 4 sets of 8 repetitions of **Tricep Lifts**.

1. Start by sitting comfortably towards the front of your chair, and your feet should be flat on the ground and underneath your hips. Keep your shoulder relaxed, back and down.

2. Put your hands on either side of the seat of the chair near your hips or on the armrests.

3. Lean slightly forward at the hips while keeping your back straight.

4. Now press through your hands, straightening your elbows and lifting your buttocks off the chair, if you can.

5. Slowly lower your buttocks back to the chair by bending at your elbows.

6. Repeat for 8 repetitions.

*Rest for 2 minutes between sets.

HIIT Workout

You will now do 30 seconds of work with 30 seconds of rest for each movement.

- jumping Jacks
- squats
- burpees
- lunges

*Rest for 2 minutes and repeat once more.

Cool-Down

1. Start by standing up tall or, if you prefer, sitting down comfortably in a chair.

2. Your feet should be placed underneath your hips.

3. Place your arms on your thighs, or let them hang to your side.

4. Look over to your left shoulder as far as you feel comfortable.

5. Hold for 30 to 60 seconds.

6. Look over to your right shoulder as far as you feel comfortable.

7. Hold for 30 to 60 seconds.

8. Carefully return your head to the starting position.

9. Bring your ear down to your shoulder; do not bring your shoulder up to your ear; leave your shoulder relaxed. Go as far as you feel comfortable.

10. To increase the stretch, place your hand on the side of your head and apply gentle pressure.

11. Hold this position for 30 to 60 seconds.

12. Repeat the stretch on each side 2 to 3 times.

13. Raise your arms straight up in front of you, parallel to the floor.

14. Now, bring your arms out to the side, pulling as far back as you can and squeezing your shoulder blades together while keeping your posture upright.

15. If you have difficulty holding your arms at 90 degrees (or parallel to the floor), you can hold your arms lower (45 degrees).

16. Hold this position for 30 to 60 seconds.

17. Sit towards the front of your chair with your shoulders relaxed, back and down. Keep your feet flat on the floor and slightly out in front of you. Your hands can be on your lap.

18. Put one of your hands behind your head, and your other hand can be left hanging straight beside you.

19. Slowly lean down to the side with the straight arm until you can feel a stretch on the opposite side. (If it is uncomfortable to

place your hand on your hand behind your head, you can keep it on your lap).

20. Stand up with your feet together and arms at your sides.

21. Breathe in and step your left foot back about 3 to 4 feet while keeping your right foot forward. Your right knee should be directly above your right ankle.

22. Turn your left foot at a 45-degree angle, making sure that your left heel is grounded.

23. Pivot your hips to face the side of your mat, aligning your torso over your pelvis.

24. Breathe out and lift your arms to the sides, parallel to the floor. Your palms should face down.

25. Look over your right fingertips, maintaining a steady focus.

26. Keep your right knee bent and your left leg straight, holding the pose for 20 to 30 seconds while breathing deeply.

27. To release the pose, breathe in and lower your arms back to your sides. Step your left foot forward to meet your right foot.

28. Perform the pose on the opposite side by stepping your right foot back and repeating the steps.

45-Minute Lower Body Workout

Warm-up

1. Start by standing up tall, and your feet should be underneath your hips. Keep your shoulder relaxed, back and down, with your arms by your side.

2. Raise your arms out to the sides and overhead and jump or step your feet out so they're slightly more than shoulder-width apart.

3. Without pausing, quickly bring your arms back down to your side and your feet together.

4. Repeat for 30 to 60 seconds.

5. Rest for 1 minute and repeat.

6. Place your hands on your hips.

7. Gently rotate your hips in a clockwise direction. Start with small circles, and as you progress through your repetitions, expand them.

8. Rotate for 12 to 15 repetitions.

9. Return to the center and repeat in an anticlockwise direction.

10. Stand up tall. Your feet should be about shoulder-width apart. Keep your shoulder relaxed, back and down, with your arms by your side.

11. Gently bend down until your hands touch the flow.

12. Carefully and slowly walk your hands forward until you get into a plank position or as far as comfortable.

13. Pause for a second, then walk your hands back toward your feet.

14. Return to standing.

15. Continue for 30 to 60 seconds.

The Workout

Perform 3 sets of 12 **Squats**.

1. Start by standing up tall next to a chair or counter if you need support. Keep your shoulders relaxed, back and down.

2. Your feet should be shoulder-width apart, with your toes either facing forward or slightly outwards.

3. You can hold onto the chair for support or raise your arms in front of you.

4. Activate your midline carefully, bend your hips, and sit back as you would if you were to sit on a chair.

5. As you sit back, keep your chest up and your core tight; aim to go to 90 degrees or slightly lower.

6. As you stand back up, put equal weight through both legs, ensuring your feet stay flat on the floor throughout.

7. Make sure your knees stay in the line of your toes; they don't go forward past your toes, and they aren't moving inward throughout the exercise.

*Rest for 90 seconds between sets.

Perform 3 sets of 6 repetitions each. **Lateral Lunge**.

1. Start by standing tall. Your feet should be about hip-width apart. Keep your shoulders relaxed, back and down, with your hands on your hips or clasped in front of your chest.

2. Carefully take a wide step to your right with your right foot. Keep your left leg straight as you begin to bend your right knee.

3. As you step to the side, push your hips back and lower your body toward your right knee. Make sure that your right knee stays aligned with your right foot and does not extend past your toes.

4. Keep your back straight by keeping your chest up throughout the movement. Try to avoid rounding your back.

5. Lower your body until your right thigh is parallel to the ground or as low as you can comfortably go. Hold this position for one breath.

6. Push through your right foot to return to the starting position, and activate your glutes and leg muscles as you stand up.

7. Once you've completed your repetitions on the right side, repeat the movement on your left side by stepping to the left and bending your left knee while keeping your right leg straight.

*Rest for 90 seconds between sets.

Perform 3 sets of 8 **Kettlebell Deadlift**.

1. Place the kettlebell on the floor between your feet. You should be facing the kettlebell.

2. Bend forward at your hips and bend your knees slightly. Keep your back straight and your chest up as you lower your body toward the kettlebell.

3. Reach down and take hold of the kettlebell handle with both hands, making sure that you have a firm grip.

4. Before you lift, activate your midline and core muscles to stabilize your body.

5. Push through your heels and extend your hips and knees simultaneously to lift the kettlebell. Keep the kettlebell close to your body as you stand upright.

6. At the top of the lift, stand tall with your shoulders back and chest forward. The kettlebell should be hanging in front of your thighs.

7. To lower the kettlebell, bend your hips first, then bend your knees. Keep your back straight as you guide the kettlebell back down toward the floor.

8. Reset your position and repeat the movement.

*Rest for 2 minutes between sets.

Perform 3 sets of 12 **Calf Raises**.

1. Start by standing up tall next to a chair or counter if you need support. Keep your shoulders relaxed, back and down.

2. Your feet should be hip-width apart.

3. Keep your knees straight and hold onto the chair for support if needed.

4. Come up onto your toes and raise your heels off the floor.

5. Hold this position briefly before lowering yourself back down.

6. Repeat 12 repetitions

*Rest for 2 minutes between sets.

Perform 3 sets of 8 **Side Leg Raises**.

1. Begin by lying on your side on a mat or flat surface with your knees bent and feet flat on the floor, hip-width apart. You can either rest your head on your arm or place a cushion under your head to make yourself comfortable.

2. Keep your body in a straight line from your head to your feet, with your legs stacked on top of each other.

3. Bend your bottom leg at your knee while keeping it flat on the ground to keep you stable. You can also keep it straight if you prefer.

4. Keep your top leg straight as you slowly lift it up toward the ceiling. Activate your glutes and midline as you raise your leg.

5. Lift your leg till it is about 45 degrees off the ground or as high as you feel comfortable. Hold this position for a breath while making sure your body remains in a straight line.

6. Slowly lower your leg back down to the starting position.

7. Repeat 8 repetitions on one side, then swap sides and repeat on the other.

*Rest for 30 minutes between sets.

HIIT Workout

Perform each exercise for 30 seconds, followed by 1 minute of rest. Repeat the circuit once.

- marching in place
- calf raises
- push-ups
- squats
- kettlebell Deadlift

*Rest for 1 minute and repeat once more.

Cool-Down

1. Start by standing up tall next to a chair or counter for support. Your feet should be underneath your hips. Keep your shoulder relaxed, back and down, with your arms by your side.

2. Place one foot behind you, making sure your toes are facing forward throughout the exercise.

3. Now, bring your front knee towards the chair, ensuring that your heels remain in contact with the floor at all times.

4. Hold this position for 30 to 60 seconds and then change legs.

5. Take one large step out to the side and face your toes outwards.

6. Shift your weight to one side, bending that knee. You will feel a stretch on the inner thigh of the straight leg.

7. Hold this position for 30 to 60 seconds and then change legs.

8. Sit down in your chair.

9. Straighten both of your legs in front of you and cross one leg over the other leg.

10. In a slow and controlled way, slide your heel up your shin until over the kneecap.

11. Now bend your opposite leg up, keeping your back straight and placing your hands on your shins.

12. Stay in this position, and to add a little more stretch, you can lean forward, keeping your chest up and your shoulders parallel to the floor.

13. Hold this position for 30 to 60 seconds and then change legs.

14. Lift one leg up to your chest, bending at the knee, and hug your leg.

15. Hold this position for 30 to 60 seconds and then change legs.

16. Get into a kneeling position on your yoga mat with your big toes touching and knees spread apart about hip-width distance.

17. Breathe out and sit back on your heels, allowing your hips to rest toward your heels.

18. Breathe out and extend your arms forward, resting your forehead on the mat. Alternatively, you can also place your arms alongside your body with palms facing up.

19. Allow your shoulders to soften and relax into the pose.

20. Take slow, deep breaths, feeling the stretch in your back and hips as you relax deeper into the pose.

21. Stay in this pose for 30 seconds to a few minutes, depending on your comfort level.

22. To come out of the pose, gently lift your head off the mat and walk your hands back towards your body, coming back to a seated position.

45-Minute Full-Body Workout

Warm-up

1. Start by standing up tall, and your feet should be underneath your hips. Keep your shoulder relaxed, back and down, with your arms by your side.

2. Gently squat down by bending your knees and lowering your body into a squat position; place your hands on the floor in front of you.

3. Walk your feet back while keeping your hands on the ground. Your body should be in a straight line from your head to your heels (this is the plank position).

4. If you are able to, carefully lower your body towards the ground by bending your elbows and doing one push-up.

5. Walk or jump your feet back toward your hands to return to the squat position.

6. Stand or jump up as you reach your hands overhead.

7. Return to the starting position.

8. Repeat for 30 to 60 seconds.

9. Rest for 1 minute.

10. Begin marching by lifting your right knee up towards your waist. Try to keep your knee in line with your hip.

11. As you lift your knee, swing your left arm forward and your right arm back. This will create a marching rhythm.

12. Lower your right leg and lift your left knee while swinging your right arm forward and your left arm back.

13. Continue alternating legs and arms for 30 to 60 seconds.

14. Gently shrug your shoulders up towards your ears.

15. Roll them back down as you squeeze your shoulder blades together.

16. Roll them towards the front and back up towards your ears.

17. Repeat for 10 rotations.

18. Roll them in the opposite direction.

19. Place your hands on your hips.

20. Gently rotate your hips in a clockwise direction. Start with small circles, and as you progress through your repetitions, expand them.

21. Rotate for 12 to 15 repetitions.

22. Return to the center and repeat in an anticlockwise direction.

23. Raise your arms out to the side of you at shoulder height. Your palms should be facing downward.

24. Keeping your arms straight, swing both arms towards each other until they cross in front of your chest.

25. Swing them out to your side again. Repeat this, alternating between which arm is on top of the other during crossover.

26. Repeat for 20 repetitions.

27. Gently bend down until your hands touch the flow.

28. Carefully and slowly walk your hands forward until you get into a plank position or as far as comfortable.

29. Pause for a second, then walk your hands back toward your feet.

30. Return to standing.

31. Continue for 30 to 60 seconds.

32. Rest for 1 minute and repeat.

The Workout

Perform 3 sets of 8 repetitions on each side. **Bird Dogs**.

1. Begin by getting on your hands and knees on the floor. Use a yoga mat to keep you comfortable. Place your hands directly under your shoulders and your knees under your hips.

2. Activate your abdominal muscles to stabilize your torso and keep your back flat and your spine in a neutral position.

3. Slowly reach your right arm forward, extending it straight in front of you at shoulder height. At the same time, extend your left leg straight back, keeping it in line with your body and parallel to the floor.

4. Pause for a breath, focusing on your balance.

5. Return to your starting position by lowering your right arm and left leg back to the floor so that you are on all fours again.

6. Repeat the movement by extending your left arm forward and right leg back, following the same process.

7. Continue to alternate between sides for the stipulated amount of repetitions.

*Rest 90 seconds between sets.

Perform 3 sets of 8 **Kettlebell Swings**.

1. Start by standing tall. Your feet should be about shoulder-width apart. Keep your shoulders relaxed, back and down, with your arms by your side. The kettlebell should be placed on the ground in front of you. Your toes should be facing outwards slightly.

2. Bend at your hips and knees as you lower your body. Your back should be flat, and your midline should be activated. Take hold of the kettlebell handle with both hands with your palms facing towards you.

3. Carefully pull the kettlebell slightly back between your legs and allow it to rest between your inner thighs. This is your starting position.

*Rest 2 minutes between sets.

Perform 3 sets of 15 repetitions: **Crunch**.

1. Begin by lying on your back. Use a yoga mat to keep you comfortable. Bend your knees and keep your feet flat on the ground with your heels 12 to 18 away from you.

2. Place your hands behind your head for support. You will keep this position throughout the exercise.

3. Breathe out as you activate your midline and bring your chin slightly towards your chest. Curl your torso towards your thighs.

4. Keep your neck relaxed and keep your chin towards your chest. Your feet and lower back stay on the floor throughout the whole movement. Continue to curl yourself up until your upper back lifts off the floor.

5. Hold this position briefly.

6. Return to your starting position by gently curling back down.

7. Repeat for 15 repetitions.

*Rest 45 seconds between repetitions.

Perform 3 sets of 3 repetitions: **Inchworms**.

1. Start by standing tall. Your feet should be about shoulder-width apart. Keep your shoulders relaxed, back and down, with your arms by your side.

2. Bend at your waist and reach down towards the ground, trying to keep your legs straight. If you can't touch the ground, it's okay to bend your knees slightly.

3. Place your hands on the ground in front of you and walk them forward until you are in a plank position (hands under your shoulders, body in a straight line).

4. Keep your core engaged to ensure your body stays straight and stable.

5. Take small steps to walk your feet towards your hands, keeping your legs as straight as possible. This will bring you back into a standing position.

6. Once you are back in the starting position, bend forward again and repeat the movement.

7. Repeat for 3 repetitions.

*Rest 45 seconds between repetitions.

Perform 3 sets of 5 repetitions: **Squat to Overhead Press**.

1. Start by standing up tall. Keep your shoulders relaxed, back and down. Hold two dumbbells at shoulder height with your palms facing forward and elbows bent.

2. Your feet should be shoulder-width apart, with your toes either facing forward or slightly outwards.

3. Lower your body into a squat by bending at your hips and sitting back as you would if you were to sit on a chair. Make sure your knees stay in the line of your toes. They don't go forward past your toes, and they aren't moving inward throughout the exercise.

4. As you sit back, keep your chest up and your core tight; aim to go to 90 degrees or slightly lower.

5. As you reach the bottom of the squat (thighs parallel to the ground or lower), transition to the overhead press position by keeping the weights at your shoulders.

6. As you stand back up, put equal weight through both legs, ensuring your feet stay flat on the floor throughout while lifting the weights overhead by extending your arms fully overhead as you stand upright, ensuring your elbows are locked at the top.

7. Lower the weights back to shoulder height as you prepare for the next squat.

8. Repeat for 5 repetitions.

*Rest for 2 minutes between sets.

Cool-Down

1. Begin by sitting on the floor with your legs stretched out in front of you.

2. Carefully bend your knees and bring the soles of your feet together. Drop your knees out to your sides. Your feet should be pulled in close to your groin.

3. Take hold of your feet with your hands while keeping your back straight.

4. Sit up tall, activate your midline, and make sure your shoulders are relaxed and away from your ears.

5. Breathe and relax by taking several deep breaths, gently pressing your thighs towards the floor to deepen the stretch.

6. Hold this position for 30 seconds to 1 minute, breathing deeply throughout.

7. To release this pose, slowly let go of your feet and extend your legs back out in front of you.

8. Now lie down with your legs extended behind you, feet hip-width apart.

9. Place your elbows directly under your shoulders and keep your forearms on the ground; your fingers should be pointing forward.

10. Keep your body aligned by keeping your legs and feet together and pressing the tops of your feet into the floor.

11. Gently lift your chest off the ground while keeping your pelvis and lower body on the floor.

12. Lengthen your spine and activate your back muscles, drawing your shoulder blades down and together, and lengthen your neck.

13. Keep your gaze forward and keep looking slightly ahead; your chin should be parallel to the floor.

14. Take deep breaths, holding the pose for 30 seconds to 1 minute, feeling the stretch in your lower back.

15. When you are ready to release the pose, you can slowly lower your chest back down to the ground.

16. Place your hands directly under your shoulders and your knees under your hips.

17. As you breathe in, arch your back, lift your tailbone, and drop your belly towards the floor. Gaze slightly upward, opening your chest. This is a cat.

18. As you breathe out, round your back towards the ceiling, tucking your chin to your chest and pulling your belly button towards your spine. This is a cow.

19. Continue to alternate between Cow Pose and Cat Pose, inhaling as you move into Cow and exhaling as you move into Cat.

20. Perform this for 5-10 cycles, synchronizing your breath with your movements.

21. After your last Cat Pose, return to a neutral tabletop position and take a few deep breaths.

Chapter 9:

Nifty Nutrition

Now that you have your exercise regime dialed in and you have taken care of your movement goals, it is time to look at your nutrition. Your nutrition not only provides you with energy, but it also helps you recover, allowing you to go about your days energized.

Let's look at the basics of nutrition, beginning with calories and macronutrients.

Calories and Macronutrients

Calories are a unit of measurement that tells us how much energy the food that we consume provides us. Our bodies need a set amount of calories to keep us functioning optimally which includes maintaining body temperature, supporting physical activity, and carrying out metabolic processes.

Calories are further broken down into macronutrients, and macronutrients are nutrients that our bodies require in large amounts. There are four main macronutrients:

- protein
- carbohydrates
- fats

Protein

Every gram of protein equals four calories. Protein turns into amino acids when broken down by our bodies and these amino acids are used for various bodily functions.

Amino acids help to create new proteins within your body and they are also used to build and repair tissues and muscles. They provide structure to hair, skin, nails, and organs, as well as your body's cell membrane.

They also play an important role in maintaining our pH balance as well as creating enzymes and hormones (Streit, 2021).

Sources of Protein

Adding a variety of protein sources into your diet can improve your overall health and well-being. Here's a comprehensive list of healthy protein sources, including both animal and plant-based options.

1. **Chicken breast**
   - A lean source of protein, chicken breast offers about 26 grams of protein per 3-ounce serving, making it a popular choice for building and maintaining muscle.

2. **Salmon**
   - Rich in omega-3 fatty acids, salmon not only provides around 22 grams of protein per 3-ounce serving but also supports heart health.

3. **Eggs**
   - Whole eggs are a complete protein source, containing about 6 grams of protein each, along with essential vitamins and minerals.

4. **Greek yogurt**
    - With approximately 20 grams of protein per cup, Greek yogurt is an excellent dairy option that also contains probiotics for gut health.

5. **Lentils**
    - A fantastic plant-based protein source, lentils provide about 18 grams of protein per cooked cup and are high in fiber, making them good for digestion.

6. **Quinoa**
    - This grain is unique for being a complete protein, offering 8 grams of protein per cooked cup, along with a wealth of nutrients.

7. **Chickpeas**
    - With about 15 grams of protein per cooked cup, chickpeas are versatile legumes that can be used in various dishes, contributing to both protein intake and fiber.

8. **Tofu**
    - A staple in plant-based diets, tofu contains around 20 grams of protein per cup and can absorb flavors well, making it a versatile ingredient.

9. **Almonds**
    - Nuts are great snacks, and almonds provide about 6 grams of protein per ounce, along with healthy fats that support heart health.

10. **Cottage cheese**
    - With approximately 28 grams of protein per cup, cottage cheese is low in fat and an excellent choice for a post-workout snack.

Carbohydrates

One gram of carbohydrates is the equivalent of four calories.

Our bodies convert carbohydrates into glucose. The main function of carbohydrates in our diets is to provide us with energy for our brain, central nervous system, and red blood cells. It is also stored as energy in our muscles and livers should we require it later on. Carbohydrates contain fiber, which helps with digestion and promotes healthy bowel movements, it also helps you to feel fuller for longer (Streit, 2021).

Sources of Carbohydrates

Carbohydrates provide essential fuel for daily activities. Here is a list of carbohydrate sources, focusing on vegetables, healthy grains, and fruits that not only nourish but also contribute to overall well-being.

1. **Quinoa:** Quinoa is a nutrient-dense whole grain that is gluten-free and high in protein. It contains essential amino acids and offers a good source of fiber.

2. **Oats:** Oats are a fantastic source of soluble fiber, known for their ability to lower cholesterol levels. They provide long-lasting energy and can be enjoyed as oatmeal or in baked goods.

3. **Brown rice:** Brown rice is a whole grain that retains its bran and germ, making it a healthier option compared to white rice. It provides important minerals and maintains high fiber content.

4. **Sweet potatoes:** Sweet potatoes are rich in vitamins, particularly vitamin A. They are a good source of complex carbohydrates and fiber, leading to steady energy release.

5. **Lentils:** Lentils are legumes packed with protein and fiber. They offer complex carbohydrates and can help regulate blood sugar levels, making them a smart choice for a balanced diet.

6. **Spinach:** Spinach is a leafy green vegetable loaded with vitamins and minerals. While low in calories, it contains carbohydrates that provide energy, particularly when consumed in larger quantities.

7. **Bananas:** Bananas are well-known for their potassium content and are a great source of quickly digestible carbohydrates, making them a favorite snack both before and after workouts.

8. **Berries:** Berries, such as strawberries, blueberries, and raspberries, are low in calories and high in fiber. They offer natural sweetness along with antioxidants that promote health.

9. **Whole wheat bread:** Whole wheat bread made from whole grains retains more nutrients than white bread. It provides carbohydrates along with fiber, making it a better option for sustaining energy levels.

10. **Carrots:** Carrots are a crunchy vegetable that is rich in beta-carotene and fiber. They offer a sweet taste while providing complex carbohydrates that are beneficial for energy.

Fats

One gram of fat is the equivalent of nine calories. Fats are essential to maintain our cell membrane health and to help transport and promote the absorption of the fat-soluble vitamins K, E, D, and A.

Fats can also be used as an energy source and insulate and protect your organs (Streit, 2021).

Sources of Healthy Fats

These fats provide energy, support cell growth, and help your body absorb nutrients. Here's a list of excellent sources of healthy fats to consider adding to your meals.

1. **Avocados:** Rich in monounsaturated fats, avocados can promote heart health and are packed with vitamins and minerals.

2. **Nuts:** Almonds, walnuts, and Brazil nuts are great sources of healthy fats, fiber, and protein, making them perfect snacks.

3. **Seeds:** Chia seeds, flaxseeds, and pumpkin seeds contain omega-3 fatty acids and other nutrients that benefit heart and brain health.

4. **Olive oil:** Extra virgin olive oil is known for its antioxidant properties and is a staple in Mediterranean diets; it's beneficial for heart health.

5. **Fatty fish:** Salmon, mackerel, and sardines are high in omega-3 fatty acids, which can reduce inflammation and support heart function.

6. **Coconut oil:** Though high in saturated fats, coconut oil is made up of medium-chain triglycerides, which can be converted into immediate energy.

7. **Dark chocolate:** In moderation, dark chocolate with a high cocoa content can provide healthy fats along with antioxidants.

Remember to enjoy them in moderation to reap the maximum benefits while maintaining a balanced diet.

Simple, Tasty Treats

Breakfast

Baked Blueberry Oatmeal

Time: 1 hour

Serving size: 10 people

Prep time: 50 minutes

Cook time: 10 minutes

Nutritional facts/info per serving:

Calories	184Kcal
Carbs	28g
Fat	6g
Protein	5g

Ingredients

- ¼ teaspoon salt
- 1 teaspoon ground cardamom
- 1 teaspoon baking powder
- 1 tablespoon vanilla extract
- 1 tablespoon grated lemon zest

- 2 tablespoons unsalted butter, melted
- 2 ½ cups old-fashioned rolled oats
- 1 ½ cups whole milk
- 2 large eggs, lightly beaten
- ¼ cup dark brown sugar plus 2 tablespoons, divided
- 2 cups fresh *or* unthawed frozen blueberries
- 3 tablespoons lemon juice

Instructions

1. Preheat your oven to 375 °F.
2. Lightly coat a 7-by-11-inch baking dish with cooking spray.
3. Mix together your oats, milk, eggs, 1/4 cup brown sugar, melted butter, vanilla, lemon zest, lemon juice, cardamom, baking powder, and salt in a large bowl until combined.
4. Gently stir in the blueberries until they are evenly distributed.
5. Place the mixture into the prepared baking dish; sprinkle evenly with the remaining 2 tablespoons of brown sugar.
6. Bake until golden brown and set. This should take about 40 minutes.
7. Let the oats cool for at least 10 minutes or up to 30 minutes.
8. Serve warm or at room temperature.

Spinach Omelet

Time: 10 minutes

Serving size: 1 person

Prep time: 0 minutes

Cook time: 10 minutes

Nutritional facts/info per serving:

Calories	255Kcal
Carbs	3g
Fat	19g
Protein	17g

Ingredients

- 1 teaspoon extra-virgin olive oil
- 1 teaspoon chopped fresh dill
- 2 tablespoons shredded Cheddar cheese
- 2 large eggs
- 1 cup spinach

Instructions

1. Using a small bowl, whisk the eggs together.
2. Heat the oil in a small nonstick skillet over medium-high heat and tilt the pan to coat it evenly.
3. Pour the eggs and immediately stir with a rubber spatula for 5 to 10 seconds. Then, push the cooked portions of the egg at the edge toward the center, tilting the pan to allow the uncooked egg to fill in around the edges. Continue to cook until the egg is

almost set, and the bottom is lightly golden; and this should take about 1 minute.

4. Remove the egg from the heat and top half the omelet with spinach and Cheddar. Place the other half over the filling.

5. Slide the omelet onto a plate and sprinkle dill on top.

Red Berry Smoothie

Time: 10 minutes

Serving size: 4 people

Prep time: 10 minutes

Cook time: 0 minutes

Nutritional facts/info per serving:

Calories	91Kcal
Carbs	17g
Fat	1g
Protein	5g

Ingredients

- 1 ½ cups fresh sliced strawberries
- ½ cup fresh red raspberries
- 1 (6-ounce) container of fat-free strawberry yogurt
- 1 cup fat-free milk
- 1 cup small ice cubes or crushed ice

Instructions

1. Combine yogurt, milk, and fruit in a blender.
2. Cover and blend until smooth.
3. Add ice; cover and blend until almost smooth.

Lunch

Couscous and Salmon Salad

Time: 10 minutes

Serving size: 1 person

Prep time: 10 minutes

Cook time: 0 minutes

Nutritional facts/info per serving:

Calories	464Kcal
Carbs	35g
Fat	22g
Protein	35g

Ingredients

- 2 tablespoons white-wine vinaigrette, divided
- 2 tablespoons crumbled goat cheese (1/2 ounce)
- ¼ cup sliced cremini mushrooms

- ¼ cup cooked Israeli couscous, preferably whole-wheat
- 4 ounces cooked salmon
- ¼ cup sliced dried apricots
- ¼ cup diced eggplant
- 3 cups baby spinach

Instructions

1. Using a small skillet, coat it with cooking spray and heat over medium-high heat. Add the mushrooms and eggplant and cook whilst stirring.
2. Keep stirring until the mushrooms and eggplant are lightly browned and juices have been released; and this should take 3 to 5 minutes. Remove from heat and set aside.
3. Toss spinach with 1 tbsp. Plus 1 tsp. Vinaigrette and place on a 9-inch plate.
4. Toss couscous with the remaining 2 tsp. Vinaigrette and place on top of the spinach.
5. Place the salmon on top.
6. Top with the cooked vegetables, dried apricots, and goat cheese.

Chicken Cobb Salad

Time: 5 minutes

Serving size: 1 person

Prep time: 5 minutes

Cook time: 0 minutes

Nutritional facts/info per serving:

Calories	410Kcal
Carbs	17g
Fat	22g
Protein	35g

Ingredients

- ½ hard-boiled egg, chopped
- ¼ cup chopped tomato
- ¼ cup chopped cucumber
- ¼ cup no-salt-added cannellini beans drained and rinsed
- ¼ cup sliced white button mushrooms
- 2 cups chopped romaine lettuce
- 2 tablespoons bottled blue cheese dressing
- 3 ounces grilled or roasted chicken breast, cut into cubes or strips

Instructions

1. Place lettuce in a medium bowl. Add 1 tbsp. Dressing; as you toss, it will coat the lettuce.
2. Arrange tomato, cucumber, mushrooms, chicken, egg, and beans in rows atop the lettuce.
3. Drizzle with the remaining 1 tbsp. Dressing.

Broccoli and Ham Baked Potato

Time: 10 minutes

Serving size: 1 person

Prep time: 10 minutes

Cook time: 0 minutes

Nutritional facts/info per serving:

Calories	298Kcal
Carbs	41g
Fat	19g
Protein	7g

Ingredients

- 1 tablespoon plain, nonfat Greek yogurt
- 1 6-ounce russet potato, baked
- ½ cup small broccoli florets
- 3 tablespoons diced lower-sodium ham
- ¼ cup finely shredded reduced-fat Cheddar cheese

Instructions

1. In a small microwave-safe bowl, cook broccoli until just tender.
2. Heat diced ham.
3. Top the potato with ham, broccoli, yogurt, and cheese.

Dinner

Tofu Curry

Time: 40 minutes

Serving size: 4 people

Prep time: 10 minutes

Cook time: 30 minutes

Nutritional facts/info per serving:

Calories	555Kcal
Carbs	30g
Fat	59g
Protein	22g

Ingredients

- 1 1/2 teaspoons garam masala, divided
- 1 teaspoon salt, divided
- 3 tablespoons canola oil, divided
- 2 tablespoons cornstarch
- 1 tablespoon Madras curry powder
- 1 (14-ounce) package of extra-firm tofu, drained, pressed, and patted dry
- 1 cup chopped yellow onion

- 1 medium jalapeno pepper, stemmed and finely chopped
- 1 (1 1/2-inch) piece fresh ginger, peeled and finely chopped
- 4 cloves garlic, finely chopped
- 1 (15-ounce) can no-salt-added crushed tomatoes
- 1 cup well-stirred canned coconut milk
- 1/2 cup water
- 1 (10-ounce) package frozen peas
- 1 (5-ounce) package baby spinach
- 2 cups hot cooked brown basmati rice
- Fresh cilantro leaves and tender stems for garnish (optional)

Instructions

1. Preheat oven to 400 °F.
2. Using your hands, crumble the tofu into bite-size pieces onto a rimmed baking sheet.
3. Gently toss the crumbled tofu with cornstarch, 1 teaspoon garam masala, 1/2 teaspoon salt and 2 tablespoons oil until evenly coated. Bake for about 30 minutes, stirring once halfway, until lightly golden with crispy edges.
4. While it is baking, heat the remaining 1 tablespoon oil in a medium Dutch oven over medium heat. Add onion, jalapeno, ginger, and garlic; cook for about 5 minutes, stirring often, until softened. Stir in the curry powder and the remaining 1/2 teaspoon each garam masala and salt. Cook for 30 seconds, stirring constantly, until fragrant.
5. Stir in tomatoes and coconut milk. Bring to a simmer over medium heat; simmer for 5 minutes until flavors meld.

6. Place the mixture into a blender. Secure the lid and remove the centerpiece to allow steam to escape. Place a clean towel over the opening. Blend until smooth and creamy, about 1 minute. (Use caution when blending hot liquids.)

7. Return the pureed mixture to the pot.

8. Add the baked tofu, water, peas, and spinach. Cook over medium heat for 3 to 5 minutes, stirring occasionally, until the peas are tender and the spinach is wilted.

9. Divide the rice among the 4 bowls; top with the curry. Garnish with cilantro, if desired.

White Bean and Spinach Pasta

Time: 35 minutes

Serving size: 4 people

Prep time: 0 minutes

Cook time: 35 minutes

Nutritional facts/info per serving:

Calories	442Kcal
Carbs	65g
Fat	13g
Protein	22g

Ingredients

- ¾ teaspoon salt
- ½ teaspoon ground pepper

- 1 tablespoon lemon juice
- clove garlic, grated
- 1 (5 ounces) package baby kale
- 1 (5 ounces) package baby spinach
- 8 ounces whole-wheat penne or rigatoni pasta
- 2 ounces cream cheese
- ½ cup shredded Gruyère cheese
- ½ cup torn fresh basil leaves, plus more for garnish
- 1 (15 ounces) can low-sodium white beans, rinsed

Instructions

1. Bring a large pot of water to a boil. Add the spinach and kale and cook for 3 minutes until tender. With tongs or a slotted spoon, move the greens to a colander and rinse under cold water. Wrap in a clean towel and squeeze out as much liquid as possible. Keep the water boiling.

2. Add pasta to the boiling water and cook al dente according to package instructions.

3. While it is cooking, combine the greens, cream cheese, Gruyère, basil, lemon juice, garlic, salt, and pepper in a food processor; process until the greens are finely chopped.

4. Keep 1/4 cup of the pasta water; drain the cooked pasta and return to the pot.

5. Add the reserved water to the food processor and process until the sauce is smooth.

6. Add beans and the sauce to the pasta and stir to combine. Top with more basil, if desired.

Chicken, Leek, and Brown Rice Stir-Fry

Time: 19 minutes

Serving size: 4 people

Prep time: 8 minutes

Cook time: 11 minutes

Nutritional facts/info per serving:

Calories	398Kcal
Carbs	33g
Fat	16g
Protein	26g

Ingredients

- 1 tbsp low-salt soy sauce
- 1 tbsp red wine vinegar
- 1 tbsp olive oil
- 1 leek halved lengthways and finely sliced
- 1 red pepper deseeded and chopped
- 250g chicken breast thinly sliced
- 100g chorizo chopped
- 80g kale
- 2 x 250g pouches microwave wholegrain rice

Instructions

1. Heat the oil in a frying pan over high heat and fry the chicken for 3 mins.

2. Stir in the chorizo and cook for 2 minutes more until the chicken is lightly golden, and the chorizo has released its fat. Place the chicken and chorizo into a bowl, leaving as much oil in the pan as you can.

3. Set aside.

4. Put the leek and red pepper into the pan and cook for 2 minutes, stirring frequently until slightly softened. Add the kale and fry for 1 minute more until the leaves have just started to wilt at the edges.

5. Drizzle in the soy sauce and vinegar and add the rice, breaking up any large chunks with a wooden spoon.

6. Stir the chicken and chorizo back into the pan and toss everything together to combine.

7. Cook for 3 minutes until the rice is heated through, then serve.

Key Takeaways

- Nutrition is vital for energy and recovery, enhancing daily activity and exercise.
- Macronutrients include protein, carbohydrates, and fats, each serving unique functions in the body.
- A variety of protein sources contribute to overall health and muscle repair.
- Carbohydrates provide essential energy and support digestive health through fiber.

- Fats play a critical role in vitamin absorption and protecting organs.

Conclusion

You have taken the first steps toward a healthier, happier life filled with energy and vitality. For many of us, reaching our golden years can bring new challenges. Yet, it also provides us with insights that we might not have considered before, especially when it comes to taking care of our bodies.

As we made our way through this book, we explored various exercises designed specifically for you. Whether you have mobility issues or are managing chronic conditions, there is a way for you to move your body safely. We've looked at routines that are not only safe but also designed to strengthen your body, improve your balance, and, as a result, improve your quality of life. By adding these exercises into your daily routine, you're not simply going through the motions; you are empowering yourself to live fully and independently.

It is never too late to start moving, as there is a profound connection between physical activity and well-being. Whether you have been active all your life or are just stepping into the world of fitness, each exercise was chosen to be both impactful and achievable.

The beauty of these routines lies in their adaptability. Whether you're standing or seated, each exercise adapts to fit your individual needs and meets you where you are on your fitness journey.

But it doesn't end here. Fitness isn't a destination; it's a lifetime commitment and an investment in yourself.

Yes, we are getting older, but never forget your strength and potential. I hope you have been inspired to explore new ways of staying active. Let curiosity lead you toward new adventures and don't be afraid to challenge yourself. You are very capable.

References

ACE Fitness. (n.d.). *ACE - certified: June 2023 - aging and moving well: 10 key exercise programming tips for older adults.* https://www.acefitness.org/continuing-education/certified/june-2023/8353/aging-and-moving-well-10-key-exercise-programming-tips-for-older-adults/

Afonso, J., Brito, J., Abade, E., Gonçalo Rendeiro-Pinho, Baptista, I., Figueiredo, P., & Fábio Yuzo Nakamura. (2023). Revisiting the "whys" and "hows" of the warm-up: are we asking the right questions? *Sports Medicine, 54*(1). https://doi.org/10.1007/s40279-023-01908-y

British Journal of Sports Medicine. (2023). *Exercise and mental health: A vital connection.* https://bjsm.bmj.com/content/58/13/691

CDC. (2024, May 7). *Physical activity for older adults: An overview.* https://www.cdc.gov/physical-activity-basics/guidelines/older-adults.html

Chicken, leek & brown rice stir-fry. (n.d.). BBC Good Food. https://www.bbcgoodfood.com/recipes/chicken-leek-brown-rice-stir-fry

Cronkleton, E. (2020, May 11). *Balance exercises for seniors: 11 moves to try.* Healthline. https://www.healthline.com/health/exercise-fitness/balance-exercises-for-seniors

Dansky, L. (n.d.). *Blueberry baked oatmeal.* EatingWell. https://www.eatingwell.com/recipe/8026653/blueberry-baked-oatmeal/

Healthy dinner recipes. (n.d.). EatingWell. https://www.eatingwell.com/recipes/17947/mealtimes/dinner/

Khan Academy. (2008). *Human anatomy and physiology*. https://www.khanacademy.org/science/health-and-medicine/human-anatomy-and-physiology

Kutcher, M. (n.d.). *Exercise library for seniors*. More Life. https://morelifehealth.com/exercise-library

Loh, A. (2024, October 18). *32 healthy breakfast recipes with foods to help you lose weight*. EatingWell. https://www.eatingwell.com/gallery/12907/healthy-recipes-for-breakfast-foods-to-help-you-lose-weight/

Melone, L. (2023). *7 dynamic warm ups*. Arthritis Foundation. https://www.arthritis.org/health-wellness/healthy-living/physical-activity/other-activities/7-dynamic-warm-ups

More Life Health. (2014). *Seniors health & fitness*. https://morelifehealth.com/balance-exercise-library

Mount Sinai. (2017). *Aging changes in the bones - muscles - joints*. https://www.mountsinai.org/health-library/special-topic/aging-changes-in-the-bones-muscles-joints

National Council on Aging. (2024, May 30). *The top 10 most common chronic conditions in older adults*. https://www.ncoa.org/article/the-top-10-most-common-chronic-conditions-in-older-adults/

RunRepeat. (2017). *78 science backed benefits of weightlifting for seniors*. https://runrepeat.com/weightlifting-benefits-seniors

Seguin, R. A., Epping, J. N., Buchner, D. M., Bloch, R., & Nelson, M. E. (2003). *Strength training for older adults*.

https://www.cdc.gov/physicalactivity/downloads/growing_stronger.pdf

Seguin, R., & Nelson, M. (2003). The benefits of strength training for older adults. *American Journal of Preventive Medicine, 25*(3), 141–149. https://doi.org/10.1016/s0749-3797(03)00177-6

Streit, L. (2021, November 1). *What are macronutrients? All you need to know*. Healthline. https://www.healthline.com/nutrition/what-are-macronutrients

Thorpe, M. (2017, May 25). *How to fight sarcopenia (muscle loss due to aging)*. Healthline. https://www.healthline.com/nutrition/sarcopenia

Visaria, A. (2021, April 29). *The importance of maintaining balance as we age*. Woodside Clinic. https://www.woodsideclinic.co.uk/the-importance-of-maintaining-balance-as-we-age

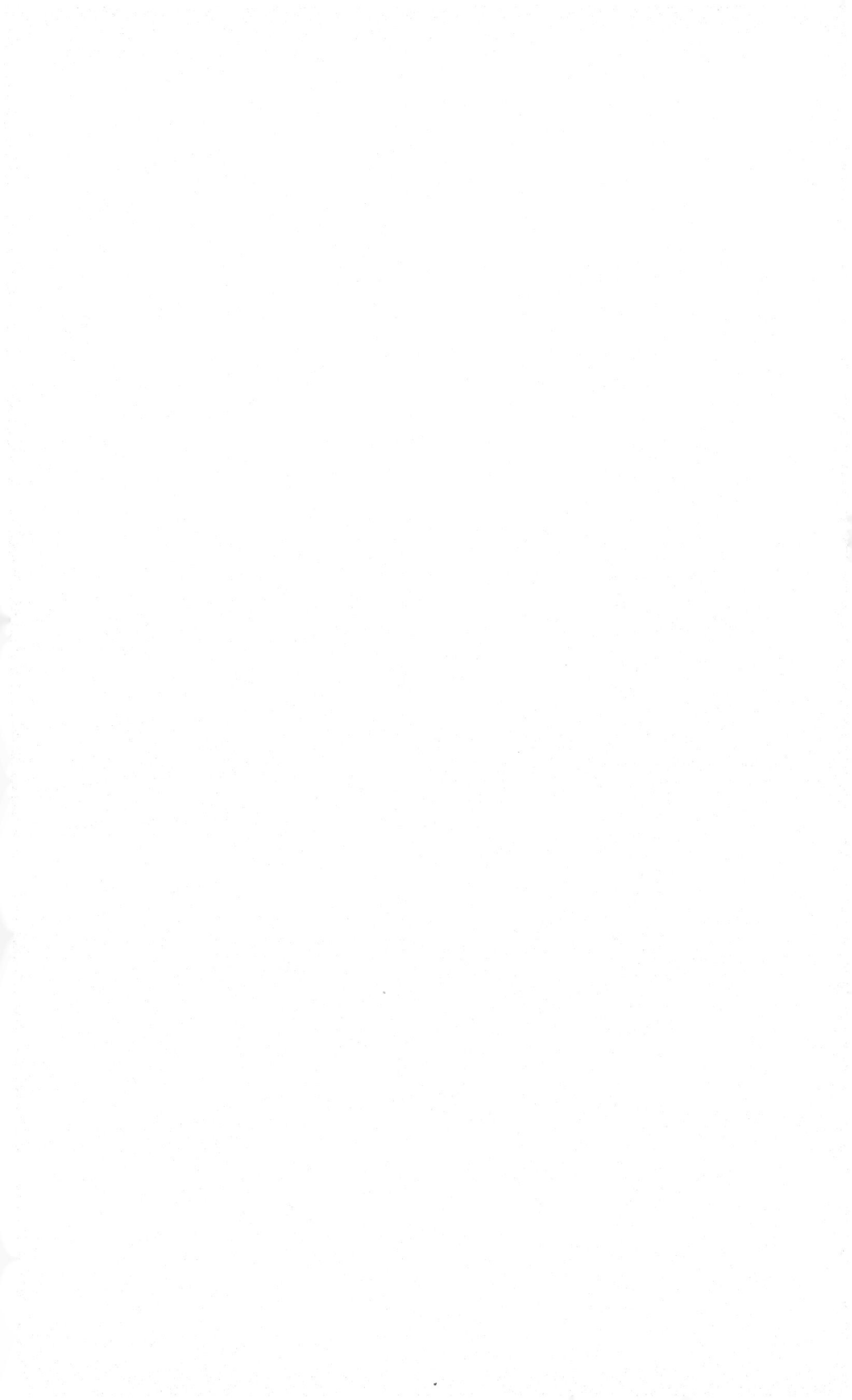

Printed in Dunstable, United Kingdom